Case Presentations in
Chemical Pathology

Titles in the series

Case Presentations in Accident and Emergency Medicine

Case Presentations in Anaesthesia and Intensive Care

Case Presentations in Arterial Disease

Case Presentations in Chemical Pathology

Case Presentations in Clinical Geriatric Medicine

Case Presentations in Endocrinology and Diabetes

Case Presentations in Gastrointestinal Disease

Case Presentations in General Surgery

Case Presentations in Heart Disease (Second Edition)

Case Presentations in Medical Ophthalmology

Case Presentations in Neurology

Case Presentations in Obstetrics and Gynaecology

Case Presentations in Otolaryngology

Case Presentations in Paediatrics

Case Presentations in Psychiatry

Case Presentations in Respiratory Medicine

Titles in preparation

Case Presentations in Urology

Case Presentations in Chemical Pathology

Martin Crook, BSc, MBBS, PhD, MRCPath
Honorary Lecturer, Chemical Pathology, University of London

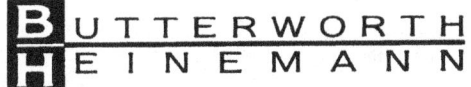

Butterworth-Heinemann Ltd
Linacre House, Jordan Hill, Oxford OX2 8DP

℞ A member of the Reed Elsevier group

OXFORD   LONDON   BOSTON
MUNICH   NEW DELHI   SINGAPORE   SYDNEY
TOKYO   TORONTO   WELLINGTON

First published 1993

British Library Cataloguing in Publication Data

A catalogue record for this book is available
from the British Library.

ISBN 0 7506 0845 5

Library of Congress Cataloguing in Publication Data

A catalogue record for this book is available
from the Library of Congress.

Composition by Scribe Design, Gillingham, Kent
Printed and bound in Great Britain by Biddles Ltd,
Guildford and King's Lynn

To my family

'that in all things He might have the pre-eminence'

Colossians 1:18

Contents

Recommendations for interpreting laboratory data

The reference ranges quoted in this book are only provided as a guide for interpreting the data presented in the case histories. The reader should always consult their own laboratories for reference range information concerning patients. The investigations discussed in this book are not necessarily exhaustive and exact details and drug dosage should always be checked in consultation with the local hospital laboratory.

Reference ranges

PLASMA

Sodium		135-145 mmol/l
Potassium		3.5-5.0 mmol/l
Chloride		95-105 mmol/l
Bicarbonate		24-32 mmol/l
Anion gap		10-16 mmol/l
Urea		2.5-7.5 mmol/l
Creatinine		0.06-0.12 mmol/l
Calcium		2.15-2.55 mmol/l
Ionized calcium		1.15-1.30 mmol/l
Magnesium		0.70-1.0 mmol/l
Phosphate		0.80-1.35 mmol/l
Urate	female	0.14-0.33 mmol/l
	male	0.20-0.43 mmol/l
Albumin		35-45 g/l
Total protein		60-75 g/l
Bilirubin, total		<20 umol/l
Bilirubin, conjugated		<3 umol/l
Aspartate transaminase (AST)		<40 U/l
Alanine transaminase (ALT)		<42 U/l
Alkaline phosphatase (adults and non-pregnant)		<250 U/l
Gamma glutamyl/transferase (GGT)	female	8-36 U/l
	male	10-55 U/l
Amylase		<200 U/l
Lactate dehydrogenase (LDH)		<210 U/l
Creatine kinase (CK)	female	<180 U/l
	male	<200 U/l
Osmolality		270-300 mmol/kg
Fasting venous plasma glucose		3.5-5.5 mmol/l
Fructosamine		1.8-2.5 mmol/l
Glycosylated haemoglobin (HbA1)		<6% of total Hb
Iron	female	11-30 umol/l
	male	14-32 umol/l
Total iron binding capacity (TIBC)		54-80 umol/l
Ferritin	female	15-300 ug/l
	male	15-200 ug/l
Serum caeruloplasmin		0.15-0.60 g/l
Ammonia venous plasma		<20 umol/l
Lactate venous fasting plasma		0.5-1.5 mmol/l
Serum carcinoembryonic antigen (CEA) non smokers		<2.5 ug/l
Serum alpha-fetoprotein (AFP) non-pregnant		<8 kU/l
Serum beta-human chorionic gonadotrophin (BHCG) non-pregnant		<4 U/l

The following fasting lipid values are rough guidelines:

Cholesterol	3.5-5.2 mmol/l
Triglyceride	0.3-2.3 mmol/l
High-density lipoprotein (HDL) cholesterol	0.9–1.8 mmol/l

SERUM HORMONES

Free thyroxine (fT4)			12-25 pmol/l
Free tri-iodothyronine (fT3)			6-13 pmol/l
Thyroid stimulating hormone (TSH)			0.20-5.0 mU/l
Growth hormone (GH)			
in response to hypoglycaemia			>20 mU/l
oral glucose suppression			<2 mU/l
Prolactin			<470 mU/l
Luteinizing hormone (LH)	male		1-7 U/l
	female	follicle	1-7 U/l
		mid-cycle	2-25 U/l
		luteal	1-4 U/l
Follicle stimulating hormone (FSH)	male		1-8 U/l
	female	follicle	1-9 U/l
		mid-cycle	2-15 U/l
		luteal	1-3 U/l
Cortisol		9 am	180-720 nmol/l
		mid-night	<220 nmol/l
Insulin fasting			<80 pmol/l
Insulin C-peptide			<450 pmol/l
Sex-hormone-binding globulin (SHBG)	male		10-45 nmol/l
	female		20-90 nmol/l
Testosterone	male		10-30 nmol/l
	female		1-3 nmol/l
Dihydrotestosterone (DHT)	male		0.9-3.0 nmol/l
	female		0.2-1.0 nmol/l
Progesterone	female	follicle	1-5 nmol/l
		luteal	>20 nmol/l
Oestradiol (E2)	male		<200 pmol/l
	female	follicle	70-380 pmol/l
		luteal	90-880 pmol/l
Parathyroid hormone (PTH)			20-65 ng/l
Calcitonin			<0.08 ug/l
Plasma adrenocorticotrophic hormone (ACTH)			20-80 ng/l
Plasma renin activity, recumbent			18-38 pmol/l/min
Plasma renin activity, ambulant			36-78 pmol/l/min
Plasma aldosterone, recumbent			140-280 pmol/l
Plasma aldosterone, ambulant			220-680 pmol/l
Vitamin D (25-hydroxycholecalciferol)			3-30 ug/l

URINE

Free cortisol	100-350 nmol/24 hour
Total calcium	2.5-8.8 mmol/24 hour
Hydroxy-methoxymandelic acid (VMA or HMMA)	<25 umol/ 24 hour
5-hydroxyindole acetic acid (5-HIAA)	<25 umol/ 24 hour
Total protein	<150 mg/ 24 hour
Porphobilinogen (PBG)	0-10 umol/l
Total porphyrins	20-330 nmol/l

MISCELLANEOUS

Fecal fat	<18 mmol/24 hour
Fecal total porphyrins	10-210 nmol/g dry weight
Erythrocyte porphyrins	0.5-2 umol/l

ARTERIAL BLOOD GASES

pH	7.33-7.45
PaO_2	90-105 mm Hg
$PaCO_2$	36-44 mm Hg

Case presentations, questions and answers

Case 1

A 79-year-old retired train driver was admitted to the geriatric ward because he was unable to cope at home following the recent death of his wife. Three years previously, non-insulin dependent diabetes mellitus (NIDDM) had been diagnosed for which he had been prescribed glibenclamide 5 mg and a diabetic diet. Otherwise, he had good health and was taking no other medication. Over the last week, however, he had described symptoms of vague weakness and muscle aching which had resolved spontaneously and had been attributed to a 'flu-like' illness. There was nothing of note in his past medical history except for an operation for an inguinal hernia 10 years previously.

On examination he was obviously overweight with a body mass index of 28.4 and blood pressure of 144/92. Otherwise examination of his systems was unremarkable, as was a resting ECG and chest X-ray. Blood was taken for a number of investigations and the following results were obtained: sodium 138 mmol/l; potassium 6.1 mmol/l; bicarbonate 27 mmol/l; chloride 105 mmol/l; urea 9.6 mmol/l; creatinine 0.17 mmol/l; random venous plasma glucose 11.2 mmol/l; and serum fructosamine 3.3 mmol/l. His serum TSH was 0.87 mU/l with a free T4 of 14.6 pmol/l and his haemoglobin was 12.8 g/dl, white cells 6.8×10^9/l and platelets 233×10^9/l. The geriatricians were a little surprised by the elevated plasma potassium, and initially thought this could be due to slight sample haemolysis or a delay in sample separation. However, a repeat plasma potassium the next day confirmed hyperkalaemia of 6.0 mmol/l. A tentative diagnosis of Addison's disease was made, but this was excluded by a normal serum cortisol response to Synacthen stimulation. Consequently, the hyperkalaemia was attributed to a chronic impairment of renal function.

Questions

1. Is renal insufficiency a likely explanation for the hyper-kalaemia?
2. What investigations could help to confirm the cause of the hyperkalaemia?
3. Suggest a likely diagnosis to account for the hyperkalaemia.

Answers

1. Chronic renal insufficiency is almost certainly not the explanation for this patient's hyperkalaemia, although admittedly it commonly causes an elevated plasma potassium in this age group. Hyperkalaemia tends to occur in end-stage chronic renal failure when the glomerular filtration rate declines to below 20 ml/min; this corresponds to a plasma creatinine concentration of about 0.35 mmol/l. This patient's plasma creatinine result clearly does not fall within this category, nor does his slightly elevated plasma urea support the notion of severe renal insufficiency.

2. The full blood count was useful in excluding causes of pseudo-hyperkalaemia, such as thrombocytosis and leucocytosis, where increased blood cells can result in a leakage of intra-cellular potassium to outside the cell. The patient was not on intravenous or oral potassium supplementation nor was he taking medication known to decrease potassium excretion. This includes potassium-sparing diuretics, for example amiloride, triamterene or spironolactone, or angiotensin-converting enzyme (ACE) inhibitors. Digoxin toxicity, beta-blockers and succinylcholine administration can all cause an efflux of potassium from cells, but again these causes are not applicable to this patient. It is also possible to exclude other causes of cellular release of potassium resulting in hyper-kalaemia from the patient's history, such as chemotherapy, crush injury, hyperkinetic activity or hyperkalaemic periodic paralysis. Admittedly, hyperkalaemia is well described in diabetic patients but usually those in ketoacidosis associated with insulin deficiency, when potassium also leaks out of the cells, but this too is not relevant to our patient. *Table 1.* lists some causes of hyperkalaemia.
   Some authors have used the plasma anion gap (the sum of the plasma sodium and potassium concentrations – the sum of

Table 1 Some causes of hyperkalaemia

Artefacts	Haemolysis
	Thrombocytosis
	Leucocytosis
Acidosis	
Cellular shifts	Malignant hyperpyrexia
	Crush syndrome
	Tumour lysis syndrome
	Periodic paralysis
	Insulin deficiency
Drugs	Intravenous/oral potassium
	Potassium-sparing diuretics
	Angiotensin converting enzyme (ACE) inhibitors
	Succinylcholine
	Beta-blockers
	Heparin
Renal	Acute or chronic renal failure
	Interstitial nephritis obstruction
	Amyloidosis
Mineralocorticoid deficiency or resistant syndromes	

the plasma chloride and bicarbonate concentrations) to help unravel the causes of hyperkalaemia, as an acidosis results in shifts of potassium out of cells. An increased anion gap in the face of a reduced plasma bicarbonate points to a metabolic acidosis as a cause of the hyperkalaemia. But this is also unlikely as this patient's plasma bicarbonate is normal as is his plasma anion gap. By this process of investigation and elimination, one has to consider either mineralocorticoid deficiency or resistant states to account for the patient's hyperkalaemia. It has already been mentioned that adrenal insufficiency manifesting as Addison's disease was reasonably excluded by the Synacthen or corticotrophin test. However, the aldosterone system also needs investigating. Indeed, early morning plasma aldosterone and renin activity were measured before rising and after four hours' ambulation. The following results were obtained:

- Plasma renin activity, recumbent, 28 pmol/l/min.
- Plasma renin activity, ambulant, 37 pmol/l/min.
- Plasma aldosterone, recumbent, 140 pmol/l.
- Plasma aldosterone, ambulant, 180 pmol/l.

3. The most likely diagnosis in the presence of these results is the syndrome of hyporeninaemic hypoaldosteronism (SHH). Note the insignificant rises in both plasma renin and aldosterone upon ambulation and low normal values in both recumbent and ambulant states. This diagnosis is made more likely by its known association with diabetes mellitus, and because this syndrome is more common in the elderly particularly if they have mildly impaired renal function. The plasma aldosterone and renin data also tend to exclude the mineralocorticoid or resistant syndromes, such as systemic lupus erythematosus, amyloidosis and pseudohyperaldosteronism. The drug history is often important when seeking an explanation for hyperkalaemia, as indomethacin (a prostaglandin synthetase inhibitor) can give a similar picture to SHH. Heparin can also cause an aldosterone deficiency. A trial of fludrocortisone, a mineralocorticoid agent, resulted in normalization of the hyperkalaemia and further supported the diagnosis of SHH.

Case 2

A 24-year-old traffic warden presented to her general practitioner complaining of infertility. She and her common-law husband had been trying for three years to have a child with no success. She had never been pregnant and was not taking any drugs. She was a non-smoker and did not like alcohol. In her medical history she had not had any previous operations or serious illnesses and she was asymptomatic, apart from a slight milky discharge from her left nipple that was worse during sexual intercourse. Furthermore, she had experienced amenorrhoea for the previous nine months. On physical examination, her blood pressure was 106/72, her body mass index was 25.1 and the general practitioner was unable to find any abnormalities, apart from the fact that she was able to express the milky discharge from her left nipple.

Blood tests were sent to the local chemistry laboratory for analysis and the following results were obtained: sodium 142 mmol/l; potassium 4.2 mmol/l; urea 5.2 mmol/l; creatinine 0.08 mmol/l; TSH 1.5 mU/l; fT4 15.5 pmol/l; FSH 2.5 U/l; LH 3.6 U/l; 17-beta oestradiol 186 pmol/l; prolactin 2131 mU/l.

Questions

1. Discuss the causes of hyperprolactinaemia.
2. What is a likely explanation for the prolactin levels seen in this patient and what further investigations should be performed to confirm this?

Answers

1. The definition of hyperprolactinaemia is controversial, partly because of methodological assay differences and also because serum prolactin concentrations in the normal population are skewed and not a gaussian distribution. Several physiological factors can cause an elevated serum prolactin, including lactation, pregnancy, sleep, stress and coitus (*Table 2*). Some authors believe that a female serum prolactin level below 400 mU/l essentially excludes pathology, and generally the higher the serum concentration the greater the likelihood that one is dealing with a prolactinoma. However, primary hypothyroidism and chronic renal failure can result in an elevation of prolactin, but both are reasonably excluded in our patient upon the basis of the biochemical tests. Many drugs can also result in elevated prolactin, including oestrogens, opiates and thyrotrophin-releasing hormone (TRH).

Table 2 Some causes of hyperprolactinaemia

Physiological
  • Pregnancy
  • Lactation
  • Coitus
  • Stress

Chronic renal failure

Hypothyroidism

Ectopic secretion from tumours

Drugs
  • Dopamine-depleting drugs
  • Dopamine-receptor blocking drugs
  • Opiates

Prolactinomas
Disorders of pituitary or hypothalamus

Since dopamine inhibits prolactin release, dopamine-depleting drugs such as reserpine and methyldopa can cause increased serum prolactin, as can dopamine-receptor antagonists such as metoclopramide, haloperidol or the phenothiazines. A number of pituitary and hypothalamic disorders can inhibit the ability of hypothalamic pathways from inhibiting the secretion of prolactin from the anterior pituitary cells, thus resulting in hyperprolactinaemia. Thus when considering a case of hyperprolactinaemia, one should also bear in mind head injuries, brain tumours and granulomatous disorders. Certain tumours, e.g. some lung carcinomas, can also release ectopic prolactin or prolactin-like substances.

Prolactinomas, which are prolactin secreting pituitary tumours, are another source of elevated serum prolactin. It has been suggested that prolactin concentrations greater than 6000 mU/l indicate a macroprolactinoma, which usually enlarges the pituitary fossa. As a rough rule of thumb, microprolactinomas (defined as tumours of less than 1 cm diameter) result in serum prolactin levels between 2000-4000 mU/l, whereas a prolactinoma often causes prolactin concentrations betwen 4000-6000 mU/l. Sometimes these tumours can be mixed with cells secreting adrenocorticotrophin or growth hormone (GH), and patients may therefore show additional features of Cushing's syndrome or acromegaly. It is also important to be aware of pseudoprolactinomas. These consist of non-functioning cells, but result in hyperprolactinaemia because they interrupt the dopamine inhibition of prolactin.

2. This patient's serum prolactin is sufficiently elevated to suggest a microprolactinoma. Other causes of hyperprolactinaemia should first be excluded as discussed above. Further investigations are necessary to confirm this. Imaging techniques, such as CAT or MRI scanning of the pituitary, may show a prolactinoma. This may also be suggested by defects in the patient's visual fields. Furthermore, pituitary reserve can be assessed by a combined pituitary function test monitoring the response of thyroid-stimulating hormone to TRH, the response of follicle-stimulating hormone and luteinizing hormone to luteinizing-hormone-releasing hormone (LH-RH) and of GH and cortisol to insulin-induced hypoglycaemia. If the prolactinoma is large, there is more likelihood of an impaired pituitary reserve. Remember, however, that care is needed in closely monitoring the patient during insulin-induced hypoglycaemia (venous blood plasma glucose below 2.8 mmol/l).

Case 3

A 61-year-old semiconscious man was admitted to casualty. He was well known to the department for frequent admissions related to ethanol abuse. On previous visits to casualty, he had admitted to drinking half a bottle of whisky per day and also to smoking 15 cigarettes per day. His speech was incoherent, his manner was aggressive and he smelt of alcohol. Physical examination showed a blood pressure of 146/92 with hepatomegaly. Blood was sent for laboratory analysis and the following results were obtained: random venous blood glucose 5.3 mmol/l; bilirubin 64 μmol/l; albumin 36 g/l; alanine transaminase 205 U/l; gamma-glutamyl transaminase 871 U/l; alkaline phosphatase 342 U/l; haemoglobin 14.5 g/dl; white cells 12.6 × 10⁹/l; platelets 131 × 10⁹/l; MCV 101fl.

Questions

1. What is the ethanol-related liver problem that this patient shows?
2. What other biochemical changes due to ethanol abuse may be shown by clinical chemistry tests?
3. Name biochemical markers that can be used to detect ethanol abuse.

Answers

1. The liver function tests are consistent with acute alcoholic hepatitis. However, routine liver function test results such as these can not clearly distinguish between alcoholic hepatitis, infectious hepatitis or cirrhosis. For this, a liver biopsy may be necessary. Nevertheless, the blood results do suggest cholestasis with an increase in alkaline phosphatase (ALP) and hepatocyte damage reflected by elevated alanine transaminase (ALT).

   Classically, there are four major groups of hepatic changes related to ethanol abuse. In the first group, there are changes in the serum liver enzymes when aspartate transaminase (AST) usually increases by more than ALT. Thus the DeRitis ratio (AST:ALT) increases to greater than 1. Serum gamma-glutamyl transaminase (GGT) also frequently increases, sometimes as high as 10 times the upper reference limit.

The second condition is fatty liver. This is associated with the previously mentioned enzyme changes, slight elevation of both serum bilirubin and alkaline phosphatase, and also hepatomegaly, nausea and anorexia. Fatty liver can be reversible or can progress to alcoholic hepatitis, as in our patient. This condition is sometimes confused with extra-hepatic cholestasis, such as gall-stones. However, useful clues to its presence, apart from a history of alcohol abuse, are that serum AST is often more elevated than ALT and serum bilirubin tends to increase more in proportion than ALP. Another useful pointer is that the serum GGT tends to be considerably elevated. Elevated serum bilirubin or prothrombin time have been used to classify the severity of this disease. Liver biopsy may show steatonecrosis and Mallory's hyaline.

Fatty liver and alcoholic hepatitis can both progress to cirrhosis, with extensive liver fibrosis, regenerating hepatic nodules, and a failure of hepatic synthetic capacity, reflected by a reduced serum albumin in the presence of elevated serum transaminases, ALP and bilirubin. Interestingly, if there is severe hepatocyte damage, the transaminases may only be slightly elevated. The cirrhosis can itself progress to hepatic failure and in some cases hepatoma.

Another important, hepatic consequence of alcohol abuse is Zieve's syndrome, which is characterised by elevated bilirubin and jaundice, hypertriglyceridaemia and haemolytic anaemia.

2. Besides abnormal liver function tests, ethanol abuse can result in many other biochemical abnormalities. Acute pancreatitis is an obvious alcohol-related complication associated with elevated serum amylase and lipase concentrations. It is rare for ethanol to elicit serious glucose intolerance, although hepatocyte damage or pancreatic damage can result in this condition. Hypoglycaemia is well described, particularly in chronically malnourished alcoholics, due to a number of factors including inhibition of glycogenolysis and potentiation of insulin activity. Although rare, alcoholic ketoacidosis can manifest as ketosis, with water and saline depletion and with comparatively normal blood glucose concentrations.

Serum immunoglobulins IgA and/or IgG levels rise in alcoholism. The explanation is not clear but might illustrate antibody production to alcoholic hyalin. Note that this patient's haematology results showed a leucocytosis, low platelet count and a macrocytosis. Alcoholics tend to show low serum folate levels and have impaired vitamin B_{12} absorption. As a result of poor nutrition, other vitamin deficiencies may be found. Iron deficiency anaemia can also be displayed as a consequence of blood loss due to gastritis, peptic ulceration or bleeding varices. However, some alcoholics show moderate iron accumulation possibly due to iron containing alcoholic beverages.

Electrolyte disturbances are common, such as hypomagnesaemia, hypocalcaemia and hypophosphataemia. A low plasma zinc concentration has also been described in some patients. The explanation of these disturbances is presumably due to poor dietary intake and/or an increased urinary excretion of these compounds.

Hormonal changes may occur, including pituitary insufficiency with impaired growth hormone, prolactin and gonadotrophin release. The latter probably explains the low levels of plasma testosterone in some alcoholics. For as yet unknown reasons, increased plasma cortisol and features of Cushing's syndrome are sometimes observed; this is being called pseudo-Cushing's syndrome.

Hyperlipidaemia, apart from that seen in Zieve's syndrome, is relatively common in alcoholics, particularly elevation of serum triglycerides. High-density lipoprotein (HDL) cholesterol also tends to be elevated, mainly HDL3. Hyperuricaemia is also associated and may sometimes result in gout. Individuals abusing alcohol are also more likely to suffer from myopathy or myositis, resulting in an elevated serum creatine kinase.

3. Biochemical markers used for ethanol abuse include an elevated serum GGT. This can be raised by only a modest alcohol consumption, due to enzyme induction in the liver. The DeRitis ratio (AST:ALT) has also been used as discussed. More recently, interest has focussed on raised serum desialylated transferrin as an indicator of ethanol abuse. Other tests being investigated include the measurement of haemoglobin-associated acetaldehyde and urinary free and conjugated ethanol, and elevated beta-hexosaminidase.

Case 4

A 21-year-old engineering student was admitted to hospital by the oncologists to begin a course of chemotherapy for a recently diagnosed testicular neoplasm. He had first noticed a testicular swelling three months previously which had slowly got larger. He had recently undergone surgery to remove his left testicle and histology had shown the presence of a teratoma. Unfortunately, a computerized tomography (CT) scan had shown the presence of para-aortic lymph node enlargement. He had previously been in good health and was a non-smoker. A chemotherapy regime was started consisting of cisplatin. Apart from episodes of vomiting, for which he was given anti-emetics, his post-chemotherapy period was unremarkable and he did not develop diarrhoea or become septic. Routine blood tests were sent to the chemistry and haematology department each day post-chemotherapy. On the third day, the following biochemistry results were obtained: sodium 135 mmol/l; potassium 3.5 mmol/l; urea 8.5 mmol/l; creatinine 0.12 mmol/l; calcium 2.10 mmol/l; phosphate 0.81 mmol/l; magnesium 0.40 mmol/l; albumin 34 g/l.

Questions

1. What is the explanation for the abnormal plasma magnesium finding?
2. What other conditions can give rise to this finding?
3. What tumour markers could be used to monitor this man's long-term progress for his testicular neoplasm?

Answers

1. This patient clearly has severe hypomagnesaemia although he was asymptomatic. It has been recognised for some time that cisplatin is a nephrotoxic drug and can result in increased loss of magnesium from the kidney due to tubular damage. The kidneys are important organs for magnesium homeostasis with only about 5% of the filtered magnesium load being excreted under normal circumstances. Our patient was given magnesium replacement, and the hypomagnesaemia resolved and did not reappear during that hospital episode. It is important

to recognise hypomagnesaemia as tetany, seizures, cardiac dysrhythmias and other electrolyte imbalances can result if it is untreated.

2. There are many causes of hypomagnesaemia in hospital patients (*Table 3*). Inadequate dietary magnesium intake or inappropriate parenteral administration can occur. Hypomagnesaemia is relatively common in alcoholism. Impaired intestinal absorption due to fistulae, inflammatory bowel disease, or resection of the intestine are well-recognised causes. Body magnesium can also be lost as a result of prolonged vomiting, sweating or nasogastric aspiration. Hormonal disorders, including diabetes mellitus, primary hyperaldosteronism and hyperparathyroidism, can all result in hypomagnesaemia. Cellular shifts of magnesium can lead to hypomagnesaemia by internal redistribution and this may occur in patients treated with insulin, those with post-myocardial infarction and in diabetic ketoacidosis. In addition to nephrotoxic drugs, such as cisplatin and aminoglycosides, renal magnesium loss can also result from diuretic therapy (usually those that also cause urinary potassium loss), renal tubular acidosis, osmotic diuresis, Bartter's syndrome and salt-losing nephropathies. The diagnosis of hypomagnesaemia is usually obvious from the plasma magnesium concentration. However, sometimes red cell magnesium can give information concerning magnesium depletion or cellular redistribution. Indeed, there has been recent interest in low red cell magnesium concentrations in post-viral fatigue syndrome. Sometimes, the magnesium loading test can be used in which a 30 mmol/l magnesium load is given intravenously in 5%

Table 3 Some causes of hypomagnesaemia

Inappropriate replacement/intake
Renal loss
  • Nephrotoxic drugs
  • Primary hyperaldosteronism
  • Renal tubular disorders
Gastrointestinal loss
  • Fistulae
  • Malabsorption
  • Diarrhoea
Alcoholism
Hypokalaemia
Acute myocardial infarction

dextrose over a 12-hour period. A 24-hour urine collection is simultaneously commenced and if more than 30% of the administered magnesium is lost in the urine, then magnesium depletion is unlikely. The association between hypomagnesaemia, hypokalaemia and also hypocalcaemia should also be remembered.

3. The tumour markers that could be used to monitor the response to therapy of this man's tumour are the beta-subunit of human chorionic gonadotrophin (beta-HCG), alpha-fetoprotein (AFP) and placental alkaline phosphatase (PlAP). Serum beta-HCG is elevated in about 75% of teratomas and is related to trophoblastic components of the teratoma. Serum levels in excess of $1 \times 10^5 IU/l$ are associated with 40% one-year mortality. Serum AFP in patients' with germ-cell tumours relates to yolk-sac elements, whereas serum PlAP can also be used for the surveillance of tumour recurrence after treatment.

Case 5

A 22-year-old secretary presented to the surgeons with abdominal pain of recent onset. She said that she was otherwise in good health and that she had only had one previous bout of abdominal pain 10 months ago that in comparison was far less severe and resolved spontaneously. She was a non-smoker and was not on any medication, except for the oral contraceptive pill. Her family history was vague as she had left home when she was 16 and had not kept to keep in touch with her family.

Unfortunately, the pain worsened and because of this a laparotomy was performed that did not reveal any abdominal abnormality. Post-operatively, her blood pressure was elevated at 156/100 but nothing else was noted upon physical examination. Post-operative biochemical tests showed: plasma sodium 129 mmol/l; potassium 3.7 mmol/l; urea 6.0 mmol/l; creatinine 0.09 mmol/l; random venous plasma glucose 3.6 mmol/l.

Upon regaining consciousness in the surgical ward, she still had severe abdominal pain and her four-hourly blood pressure measurements showed persistent hypertension. A medical opinion was sought and the medical registrar suggested the possibility of acute intermittent porphyria in view of her abdominal pain and hypertension. Urine and faeces were sent to chemistry for porphyrin determination and the following results (with normal references in parentheses) were obtained:

- Urine porphobilinogen (PBG)   198 μmol/l (0-10)
- Urine total porphyrins   5600 nmol/l (20-330)
- Faecal total porphyrins   6100 nmol/g dry weight
                                 (10-210).

Questions

1. Are these results diagnostic of acute intermittent porphyria?
2. What is the enzyme defect in acute intermittent porphyria?
3. What further biochemical tests could be performed to confirm the diagnosis?

Answers

1. The grossly elevated urine PBG is highly suggestive of an acute porphyria. The four main types of acute porphyria are PBG-synthase deficiency, acute intermittent porphyria (AIP), hereditary coproporphyria (HC) and variegate porphyria (VP). Although the registrar was correct in diagnosing an acute porphyria, the above results do not support AIP. If this had been the case, then the faecal porphyrins should have been nearly normal and certainly not as high as measured in this patient. Thus, the differential diagnosis is between VP and HC.
2. Acute intermittent porphyria is the commonest of the acute porphyrias. It occurs in about 1 in 50 000 individuals and is caused by a deficiency in PBG-deaminase (sometimes known as uroporphyrinogen-1-synthase). In keeping with PBG-synthase deficiency (a very rare acute porphyria), but unlike VP and HC, photosensitivity and skin fragility are not usually features of the disease. Varigate porphyria and HC are rarer conditions, probably with a prevalence of 1 in 250 000. The former is due to a defect in the enzyme protoporphyrinogen oxidase, and the latter is due to coproporphyrinogen oxidase deficiency.

   All acute porphyrias are inherited as autosomal dominant conditions, except for PBG-synthase deficiency which is autosomal recessive. Note that urine PBG is not expected to be elevated in PBG-synthase deficiency. Erythrocyte porphyrins are generally not increased in the acute porphyrias. Also, hyponatraemia, as was observed in this patient, is a feature of some acute porphyrias.

3. To distinguish between the two types, a more detailed analysis of individual porphyrins is needed. In VP, the predominant faecal porphyrin is protoporphyrin IX, whereas coproporphyrin III predominates in HC. A useful test for diagnosing acute porphyria is measurement of the plasma fluorescence emission peak after excitation at 405 nm. During an acute attack of AIP and HC, a plasma emission peak at 615 nm is observed, whereas in VP a characteristic peak at 624–626 nm is found. This patient was found to have VP.

The investigation of latent porphyria, i.e. asymptomatic subjects, can be difficult, and may require the help of specialized laboratories as urine and faecal porphyrins may not necessarily be grossly abnormal. Determination of PBG deaminase can be performed in erythrocytes or protoporphyrinogen or coproporphyrinogen oxidase in nucleated cells, such as lymphocytes. As these porphyrias are inherited conditions, other family members should be studied. In addition, because certain drugs can precipitate an acute attack of porphyria, a careful drug history is needed. Note that our patient was taking the oral contraceptive pill.

Case 6

A 66-year-old retired teacher presented to his general practitioner complaining of backache and tiredness. He had been reasonably well up until three months previously when he had developed a continuous aching pain in his lower back. This made bending and lifting difficult, and he also complained of feeling more 'lifeless', particularly when walking to the shops. His previous medical history was unremarkable except for a skiing accident five years previously in which he broke his left ankle. He was not taking any medication apart from paracetamol for his backache. He was a non-smoker and only drank alcohol at Christmas or New Year. Physical examination revealed little; he was normotensive and his body systems were normal. However, his doctor found a particularly tender spot on his spine and thought his complexion was pale. He arranged for blood tests and an X-ray of the tender part of the patient's spine.

The consultant chemical pathologist phoned the surgery with the blood results that afternoon, as follows: sodium 139 mmol/l; potassium 4.4 mmol/l; urea 12.5 mmol/l; creatinine 0.18 mmol/l; calcium 2.90 mmol/l; phosphate 1.7 mmol/l; albumin 34 g/l; total protein 92 g/l.

The chemical pathologist also suggested a possible diagnosis, and said other biochemistry tests were being done to confirm it.

Questions

1. What is the most likely diagnosis?
2. What biochemical tests can be used to confirm this?
3. Give causes for a serum paraprotein.

Answers

1. The history and biochemical results suggest a diagnosis of multiple myeloma. This should always be considered in an elderly patient with impaired renal function tests, hypercalcaemia, and symptoms of backpain. A myeloma is due to the proliferation of an individual clone of plasma cells.

   Note that the total serum protein in this patient was elevated; this is observed in about 50% of patients, with total serum protein concentrations sometimes as high as 150 g/l. The slightly reduced serum albumin concentration is also characteristic of multiple myeloma. However, these features are not always present. This patient's increase in serum total protein is due to the production of a paraprotein by a single clone of plasma cells. Studies have revealed that about 50% of myeloma paraproteins are of the IgG type, 23% IgA, and 20% immunoglobulin light chains, while the remainder consist of IgM, IgD or, more rarely, IgE.

2. The diagnosis of multiple myeloma is based upon three major findings: (a) the presence of a paraprotein; (b) the evidence of bone destruction, such as the classical punched-out lytic

lesions seen on bone X-rays; (c) the presence of neoplastic plasma cells in bone marrow.

It is important that both serum and urine samples should be analyzed for paraproteins, as immunoglobulin light chains can appear in urine as the Bence-Jones protein. Quantitation of serum immunoglobulins is useful as there can be a reduced synthesis of other immunoglobulins (immuneparesis). Typing and quantitation of the paraprotein by electrophoresis, immunofixation and protein staining is helpful in monitoring treatment as well as in prognosis. Serum beta$_2$-microglobulin may also be useful in monitoring patients, with high concentrations indicating a worse prognosis.

3. Paraproteins are not exclusively confined to multiple myeloma. More rarely, they have been described in other malignant conditions, such as lymphomas, chronic lymphocytic leukaemia, heavy-chain disease, soft-tissue plasmacytomas and Waldenström's macroglobulinaemia (*Table 4*). The latter is a malignant plasma cell disease with high concentrations of IgM paraprotein and with consequent elevated serum viscosity.

Several non-malignant conditions also give rise to paraproteinaemia, including monoclonal rheumatoid factor, amyloidosis, monoclonal cryoglobulins and lichen myxoedematosis. A benign variety of paraproteinaemia has been described, in which some features of multiple myeloma are present and in which there is no significant progression of symptoms, clinical signs or paraprotein amount for at least five years follow-up.

Table 4 Some causes of a serum paraprotein

Multiple myeloma
Lymphomas
Waldenstrom's macroglobulinaemia
Other malignant conditions,
    e.g. chronic lymphocytic leukaemia and plasmacytomas
Benign paraproteinaemia
Cryoglobulinaemia
Amyloidosis

Case 7

A 22-year-old bricklayer was admitted to casualty, drowsy and feeling nauseous. The history was obtained from his girlfriend. He was an insulin-dependent diabetic diagnosed eight years ago. Over the last two days, he had taken a few of days' holiday and had been out partying without taking his insulin injections. The previous day, he had started to pass large volumes of urine and to vomit, which he put down to drinking five pints of beer. Now he was also feeling drowsy and thirsty. He denied taking any drugs but smoked 20 cigarettes per day. On physical examination, he was hyperventilating, clinically dehydrated, and smelt ketotic. His blood pressure was 98/70 while his pulse was 98 beats/min. He quickly became more drowsy and lapsed into a coma. Emergency blood was taken and the following results were returned: sodium 129 mmol/l; potassium 5.8 mmol/l; chloride 94 mmol/l; bicarbonate 9 mmol/l; urea 11.4 mmol/l; creatinine 0.19 mmol/l; venous plasma glucose 45 mmol/l; phosphate 1.9 mmol/l; pH 7.23; $PaCO_2$ 26 mmHg; and PaO_2 98 mmHg. Ketones were present in blood and urine.

Questions

1. What is the most likely diagnosis?
2. Explain the biochemical findings in this patient.
3. What else can cause elevated ketones in a patient's blood or urine?
4. What other types of coma can occur in patients with diabetes mellitus?

Answers

1. This patient has diabetic ketoacidosis. This may be due to his poor insulin compliance, but can also be precipitated by infection and other disorders.
2. The biochemistry results are typical of patients with this condition. The plasma glucose concentration is high and ketones are present in both blood and urine. Prior to insulin therapy and intravenous fluid replacement, patients tend to be hyperkalaemic due to the release of intracellular potassium into the plasma, which is potentiated by the acidosis.

Similarly, hyperphosphataemia is often seen due to shifts of intracellular phosphate. Note also the hyponatraemia which is multifactorial. One explanation is the shifts of intracellular fluid into the extracellular space, thus diluting the plasma sodium in response to the hyperglycaemia which increases extracellular osmolality. Another reason is that the patient becomes sodium-depleted due to loss in vomit and urine. The low plasma chloride may be partly due to chloride loss in vomit, while the low plasma bicarbonate and raised anion gap suggest a metabolic acidosis. The blood gas results confirm an acidosis and the low blood $PaCO_2$ implies an attempt at compensation of the metabolic acidosis by hyperventilation. The plasma urea is elevated and is partly due to dehydration.

3. Increased ketone production can also occur in starvation and after an overdose of ethanol, salicylate or methanol. Ketoacidosis is not confined to diabetes mellitus. More rarely, it can be caused by a high intake of ethanol or methanol.

4. Other causes of coma in diabetes mellitus include hypogly-caemic coma and lactic acidosis. The latter can occasionally be seen in patients on biguanide hypoglycaemic agents such as phenformin, while the former is usually caused by excess of insulin or a hypoglycaemic drug. Another cause of coma in diabetes mellitus is the hyperosmolar non-ketotic (HONK) type. This is commoner in the older non-insulin dependent diabetic (type II) patient. A high blood glucose concentration (usually higher than in diabetic ketoacidosis) and highly elevated plasma osmolality is seen in these patients, and sometimes also an elevated sodium concentration. These patients appear to have adequate insulin levels to minimize ketosis although it has been suggested that the raised plasma hyperosmolality could inhibit ketone formation.

Comas in diabetic patients can also be due to more general causes, such as drug overdose, cerebral events, and other metabolic causes.

Case 8

A 12-year-old schoolboy was seen in casualty because of a three-day history of diarrhoea. No other family members had shown similar symptoms, and his parents attributed his diarrhoea to eating a kebab after school. His parents had thought that diarrhoea and vomiting would pass away quickly, but in the last few hours, he has started to complain of weakness.

On examination, he was clinically dehydrated with loss of skin elasticity and somewhat sunken eyes. He appeared drowsy and his mouth and tongue looked dry. His blood pressure on lying down was 96/60 and his radial pulse rate was 94/min. Rectal examination revealed no melaena. Blood samples were quickly sent to the laboratory and the following results were obtained: sodium 156 mmol/l; potassium 3.0 mmol/l; bicarbonate 17 mmol/l; chloride 116 mmol/l; urea 19 mmol/l; creatinine 0.13 mmol/l; random venous plasma glucose 4.2 mmol/l.

Questions

1. What is the likely explanation for the plasma sodium result?
2. Comment upon his renal function tests.
3. What are some causes of hypernatraemia that can occur in hospital patients ?

Answers

1. The patient is clearly dehydrated due to his severe bout of diarrhoea. It should be remembered that hypernatraemia is usually the result of an extracellular sodium concentration in excess relative to that of water. Both diarrhoea fluid and gastric juice have a sodium concentration of 50–70 mmol/l. To become hypernatraemic, this patient's water intake must have been insufficient to replace his water losses. Thus hypernatraemia does not necessarily mean an increase in total body sodium and, as in this patient, hypernatraemia is often due to haemoconcentration. The patient shows signs of hypovolaemia, i.e. hypotension and increased pulse rate and this would be in keeping with hypotonic fluid depletion.

Note also the hypokalaemia that is due to loss of potassium-rich diarrhoea fluid and to urinary loss as a result of the secondary aldosteronism in response to hypovolaemia. The elevated plasma chloride concentration (hyperchloraemia) is partly due to haemoconcentration, but the hypovolaemia leads to an increase of renal reabsorption of chloride and for that matter sodium ions. Excess diarrhoea fluid also results in a loss of bicarbonate and thus a low plasma bicarbonate concentration is seen. The combination of these phenomena can give rise to a hyperchloraemic acidosis as shown in this patient.

2. This patient also shows an elevated plasma urea concentration. This is largely the result of a decrease in intravascular volume which in turn has led to a decreased glomerular filtration rate (GFR). Normally, the plasma urea:creatinine ratio is about 50:1. In this patient, the ratio has been increased by a low GFR and the fact that less urea, than creatinine is being excreted in urine. In these conditions, as a result of the reduced GFR, there is increased reabsorption of urea by the renal collecting ducts. Remember that plasma urea can increase out of proportion to that of plasma creatinine due to catabolism of protein, high-protein diets and gastrointestinal bleeding.

A particular danger in such patients is the development of acute renal failure as a result of hypovolaemia secondary to gastrointestinal fluid loss. In the presence of oliguria (<400 ml/day of urine), pre-renal failure should be considered. This condition is important to recognize as treatment of the dehydration can reverse the impaired renal function. Otherwise, there may be further deterioration in renal function leading to acute tubular necrosis (ATN). Some useful biochemical tests (*Table 5*) can be used to establish whether there is pre-renal failure or ATN.

Table 5 Biochemical tests used to establish pre-renal failure or acute tubular necrosis (ATN)

Test	Pre-renal failure	ATN
Urine urea:plasma urea ratio	>10:1	<4:1
Urine osmolality:plasma osmolality ratio	>1.5:1	<1.2:1
Urine sodium concentration (mmol/l)	<10	>20

Fortunately, this patient was successfully rehydrated with intravenous fluids and thus avoided acute renal failure. Important biochemical features in acute renal failure include hyperkalaemia, hypermagnesaemia, hyperphosphataemia, metabolic acidosis and elevated plasma urea and creatinine. Remember that oliguria or near-anuria may occur in post-renal failure due to an obstructed urinary outflow.

3. The commonest cause of hypernatraemia (*Table 6*) is a negative water balance, which can be due to the following:
   (a) Loss of predominantly hypotonic fluid, as in our patient, which can be due to diarrhoea, profuse sweating, vomiting or intestinal fistulae.
   (b) The result of pure depletion of water, as can occur in fever or hyperventilation or as a result of reduced water intake, either due to inadequate intravenous replacement, disorders of the brain's thirst centre, or in patients unable to drink.

Table 6 Some causes of hypernatraemia

Water loss
 • Renal e.g. central or nephrogenic diabetes insipidus or osmotic diuresis
Gut loss
 • Diarrhoea, malabsorption
Insensible loss
 • Fever, sweating
Inappropriate intravenous sodium administration
Excess sodium ingestion
Cushing's syndrome
Conn's syndrome
Rhabdomyolysis
Essential hypernatraemia

Water depletion can also be caused by polyuria, as in diabetes insipidus (either neurogenic or nephrogenic), or by an osmotic diuresis, e.g. mannitol or glucose. More rarely, there can be water loss into cells as is seen in rhabdomyolysis or following strenuous exercise or seizures.

Essential hypernatraemia has been described. It is thought to be a hypothalamic disorder which results in a defect of osmoreceptor function. Additionally, hypernatraemia can occur in mineralocorticoid excess, e.g. Cushing's syndrome or Conn's syndrome. Furthermore, one should not forget excess salt ingestion or the intravenous administration of sodium bicarbonate or hypertonic saline.

Case 9

A 17-year-old school-girl was referred to the endocrine clinic because of primary amenorrhoea. She attended with her mother. The girl had developed breasts at the age of 13 years. She was constitutionally well, having had no previous operations and only routine childhood illnesses. She was taking no medication. There was no family history of note and she was the only child. On examination, the patient was 1.78 m tall, with good breast development but no pubic hair. The clitoris was normal, but the vagina was blind-ending and short. Palpable swellings were located in the inguinal region. There was nothing else of note on examination.

A series of investigations were performed and some of the results now follow: karyotype 46 XY; plasma testosterone 27 nmol/l; plasma oestradiol 190 pmol/l; serum FSH 21 U/l; serum LH 29 U/l.

Questions

1. What is a possible diagnosis in this individual?
2. What are the causes of male pseudohermaphroditism?
3. The patient's mother volunteered to the doctor that she herself was taking oral hormone replacement therapy because of menopausal symptoms. She felt that this was not working and wondered whether 'hormone' blood tests would be of help. What is the value of measuring serum gonadotrophins or serum oestradiol in this situation?

Answers

1. This patient was shown to have complete androgen insensitivity syndrome. Note that the phenotype was female, with no signs of virilization, yet the karyotype was 46 XY male. Furthermore, the plasma concentrations of testosterone and oestradiol fall within the male reference range and can even be slightly elevated. The presentation is typical, i.e. a young girl being seen for investigation of primary amenorrhoea. The palpable swellings were in fact testes, and it could also be shown that the ovaries, cervix, uterus and fallopian tubes were absent.

The defect occurs in the androgen receptor which either fails to bind dihydrotestosterone (DHT) or has an intracellular post-receptor abnormality. Plasma levels of DHT are usually elevated in this condition. Partial defects of androgen insensitivity syndrome have also been described. Note the elevated serum gonadotrophin levels in response to the end organ receptor defect in the testes, i.e hypergonadotrophic hypogonadonism.

2. Other causes of male pseudohermaphroditism include 5-alpha-reductase deficiency. This enzyme can be assayed in fibroblasts and converts testosterone to DHT. Post-pubertal patients with this condition have a high testosterone to DHT plasma ratio. Other causes include disorders of testosterone synthesis, such as 17-beta-hydroxysteroid dehydrogenase deficiency (plasma androstenedione is elevated and plasma testosterone is low after hCG stimulation tests) and also the 17-alpha-hydroxylase deficiency, 17–20 desmolase deficiency or 3-beta-hydroxysteroid dehydrogenase deficiency.

Do not be confused by the female pseudohermaphroditism syndromes, which include some of the congenital adrenal hyperplasia syndromes, e.g. deficiencies of 21-hydroxylase and also 11-hydroxylase. Here individuals with a 46/XX karyotype show varying degrees of external genitalia virilization i.e. a male phenotype.

3. Although the gonadotrophins LH and FSH are elevated in the menopause because of gonadal failure, they are not necessarily normalized by oestrogen replacement. Serum oestradiol levels often appear low in patients on oral oestrogen because of its conversion to oestrone in the gastrointestinal tract and liver. Thus, serum oestradiol levels have limited value in these circumstances, except perhaps to detect patient compliance. However, serum oestradiol levels in patients with oestradiol inplants may help to detect the need to replace the inplant.

Case 10

A 69-year-old retired carpenter was admitted to the surgical ward for laser therapy on an inoperable oesophageal carcinoma.

He had been unable to eat solid food and his only food intake for the last few weeks was a little milk or tomato soup. On examination, he appeared malnourished having lost about 10 Kgs in weight over the last few months and there was evidence of muscle wasting. His blood pressure was 130/78, but he had hepatomegaly, which ultrasound had suggested was compatible with hepatic secondaries. Because of his feeding problems, he was fed initially with total parenteral nutrition (TPN), in the hope that after laser therapy for his oesophageal neoplasm he would be able to resume oral eating. He was not taking any other medication. The day after beginning TPN, a blood sample was taken for biochemical monitoring and the following plasma results were observed: sodium 135 mmol/l; potassium 3.6 mmol/l; urea 3.0 mmol/l; creatinine 0.09 mmol/l; random venous plasma glucose 5.7 mmol/l; bilirubin 12 μmol/l; alanine transaminase 36 U/l; alkaline phosphatase 323 U/l; gamma-glutamyl-transferase 378 U/l; calcium 1.94 mmol/l; phosphate 0.26 mmol/l; albumin 28 g/l.

Questions

1. What could be a possible explanation for the plasma phosphate result?
2. Explain the most likely reason for the abnormal liver function tests.
3. What other possible biochemical sequelae of TPN may show as abnormalities upon biochemical monitoring?.

Answers

1. The severe hypophosphataemia could be caused by the refeeding syndrome. Upon resumption of calorie intake, there can be a redistribution of extracellular phosphate to within the cells; this is often the case when glucose is given which enters the cells and participates in glycolysis and undergoes phosphorylation. Indeed, the commonest cause of hypophosphataemia in hospital populations is the administration of intravenous glucose. Other causes of hypophosphataemia (*Table 7*) should also be considered in certain patient groups, including poor intake due to starvation, alcoholism, vomiting or malabsorption. Liver disease can

Table 7 Some causes of hypophosphataemia

Redistribution	Intravenous glucose
	Alkalaemia
	Insulin administration
	Re-feeding syndrome
Poor intake	
Post-trauma or myocardial infarction or operation	
Alcoholism	
Liver disease and also malabsorption states	
Septicaemia	
Hyperparathyroidism or PTH-related peptide release from tumours	
Osteomalacia and hypophosphataemic rickets	
Fanconi's syndrome	

also result in increased cell uptake of phosphate and although not applicable to this patient alkalaemia and insulin therapy. Increased urinary phosphate excretion can occur with diuretic therapy and also with renal tubular disorders. Parathyroid hormone has a phosphaturic action, as does parathyroid-related peptide which can be released by certain tumours. Although the hypophosphataemia in this patient is probably multifactorial, the fact that three days after initiation of parenteral feeding his plasma phosphate returned to normal supported the concept that it was the TPN that was the predominant cause.

2. Elevated alkaline phosphatase and gamma-glutamyl-transferase in the absence of jaundice suggest hepatic metastases. This would be in keeping with the clinical finding of hepatomegaly and the ultrasound findings. Other hepatic space-occupying lesions can give similar findings. However, some patients on TPN develop a fatty liver infiltration, which can be associated with intrahepatic cholestasis. Plasma bilirubin can be elevated although it is generally quite rare for clinical jaundice to be seen. Sometimes, hepatic aminotransferases are also elevated.

3. Several biochemical changes can be produced by TPN, and careful biochemical monitoring is therefore indicated in these patients. Hyponatraemia is often seen and is due to many reasons, including sodium depletion and/or water overload. If there is a water deficit, then hypernatraemia may occur. Similarly, either hyperkalaemia or hypokalaemia can occur. The former is seen in some catabolic patients while

hypokalaemia may be due to depletion as a result of insufficient intake or excess loss.

Some patients become glucose-intolerant and thus hyperglycaemic. Conversely, sudden cessation of TPN can result in hypoglycaemia. Hypercalcaemia can also be observed. This could be due to bone resorption and may be more common in immobile patients. Interestingly, hypomagnesaemia has also been documented in TPN patients for multifactorial reasons.

Long-term TPN patients are at a greater risk of trace-element deficiencies. Zinc deficiency can result in poor wound healing, dermatitis, and impaired cell-mediated immunity. Chromium deficiency can result in intolerance of glucose, lack of selenium to cardiomyopathy and myopathy, copper deficiency can result in leucopenia and anaemia and molybdenum deficiency in amino-acid intolerance. Deficiencies of both water-soluble and lipid-soluble vitamins are also possible.

Case 11

A 26-year-old waitress attended the endocrine clinic complaining of excessive facial hair growth. This had been a problem since the age of 16 and had worsened progressively so that she now needed to shave every other day. Her periods were irregular and sometimes she could go five months without menstruating. These menstrual abnormalities had been present since her menarche at 15. She smoked 10 cigarettes per day, but did not like alcohol. She was not taking any medication. She had no regular boyfriend and had never been pregnant. On examination, her blood pressure was 120/78 and she had a body mass index of 28.4. She had prominent facial hair and also acne upon her back. Examination was otherwise unremarkable with a normal pelvic examination and no signs of virilism. Some endocrine tests were performed with the following results: TSH 2.1 mU/l; fT4 16.6 pmol/l; prolactin 232 mU/l; LH 25.4 U/l; FSH 7.4 U/l; testosterone 3.4 nmol/l; SHBG 35 nmol/l; oestradiol 256 pmol/l. A 24-hour urinary free cortisol was 322 nmol/24 hr.

Questions

1. What is the most likely diagnosis?
2. Name the other causes of hirsutism. How can these be investigated biochemically?

Answers

1. This lady had polycystic ovaries (PCO). She has a typical history with longstanding irregular menses and hirsutism. This condition is also associated with obesity (as in this patient), and recent studies have found that some cases are related to insulin resistance and also lipid abnormalities. Unfortunately, there is no definitive diagnostic investigation for this condition. However, many patients have a serum gonadotrophin ratio (LH:FSH) of greater than 3:1, although caution is needed as the ratio is assay-dependent and can be invalidated by low FSH concentrations.

   Other features often include a decreased serum SHBG and slightly elevated or high normal serum testosterone concentrations. Some laboratories give a free androgen index (FAI); this is equal to the serum testosterone concentration:SHBG concentration and is expressed as a percentage. This provides an assessment of the free or unbound testosterone and can be elevated in patients with hirsutism. There may also be hyperprolactinaemia. Serum SHBG can also be lowered in the presence of androgens, with obesity and also hypothyroidism. Note also that serum oestradiol is normal, but that if measured, serum oestrone is often increased. The diagnosis can be aided by ultrasound investigation of the ovaries.
2. There are many causes of hirsutism, including racial differences and idiopathic forms. The latter is thought to be due to excessive skin responsiveness to androgen hair growth stimulation. The clinician needs to exclude other causes of hirsutism, such as Cushing's syndrome, virilizing ovarian or adrenal tumours and congenital adrenal hyperplasia (CAH). In this patient, Cushing's syndrome was considered unlikely because of the lack of typical clinical features and the normal urinary free cortisol determination. The history can be important, as a virilizing tumour or CAH may be suggested by a short history of hirsutism with evidence of virilism, e.g. voice deepening, male-pattern balding and abnormal genitalia such as

clitoromegaly. An elevated serum testosterone, over 5 nmol/l as a rough guide, should be further investigated as one of these conditions may be present. One useful test is to see whether the testosterone level is suppressed by dexamethasone, as suppression of serum testosterone would make a tumour source less likely.

Some clinicians will also measure other androgens if an adrenal tumour is being considered, such as dehydroepiandrosterone (DHEA) or its sulphate (DHEAS) which can be markedly elevated. Ovarian tumours tend to show marked elevated serum testosterone concentrations while this is often less marked (<5.0 nmol/l) in adrenal tumours.

The diagnosis of CAH is often made during childhood but there is a late-onset variety in which hirsutism occurs but not usually systemic virilism. The common form is the 21-hydroxylase deficiency CAH in which 17-hydroxyprogesterone can be measured in a random blood sample. However, because of an overlap with normal values, a short Synacthen stimulation test may be preferable. An elevated serum concentration above about 46 nmol/l is suggestive of 21-hydroxylase deficiency CAH. The rarer 11-hydroxylase variety of CAH can be similarly investigated by looking for elevated serum 11-deoxycortisol after Synacthen stimulation, whereas the 3-beta-hydroxy steroid dehydrogenase deficiency form of CAH can be likewise investigated by assaying for serum DHEA or 17-hydroxypregnenolone along with urine steroids.

Case 12

A 33-year-old male accountant attended a company health screening programme. He stated that he felt perfectly well and that he had not had any operations. He did not smoke nor was he taking any medication, although he did admit to drinking two glasses of wine per day. There was little of note in his family history except that his father had been investigated for what he thought was 'raised calcium in the blood'. Physical examination found a blood pressure of 146/86 and a body mass index of 25.6. There was nothing of note in his cardiovascular, respiratory, abdominal or nervous systems. A resting electrocardiograph and a chest X-ray were normal. Blood was taken for routine biochemistry screening and revealed the following results: sodium 136 mmol/l; potassium 4.3 mmol/l; urea 5.6 mmol/l; creatinine 0.11 mmol/l; calcium 2.82 mmol/l; phosphate 0.88 mmol/l; albumin 39 g/l; bilirubin 17 μmol/l; alkaline phosphatase 124 U/l; alanine transaminase 33 U/l; random cholesterol 5.8 mmol/l.

Questions

1. What is the albumin-corrected calcium in this patient?
2. Suggest investigations you would perform to help find an explanation for the hypercalcaemia.
3. This patient's daily urinary calcium excretion was 1.8 mmol/24 hours when his hypercalcaemia was noted. What is the most likely diagnosis?

Answers

1. The albumin-corrected plasma calcium is 2.84 mmol/l. This is based on the following formula:
   Measured plasma calcium concentration + (40 – the measured albumin concentration g/l) × 0.02.
2. When faced with a case of hypercalcaemia, it is worthwhile repeating the blood test with minimal venous stasis and without a tourniquet. A borderline elevated plasma calcium is best checked on at least two occasions to confirm the diagnosis. The plasma phosphate concentration can also be a useful test in hypercalcaemia. It is often reduced in cases of primary hyperparathyroidism or due to the release of parathyroid hormone-like substances. Determination of plasma alkaline phosphatase may give additional information, as this enzyme can sometimes be elevated in primary hyperparathyroidism as well as in instances of bone metastases resulting in hypercalcaemia. A mild hyperchloraemic acidosis may also sometimes occur in primary hyperparathyroidism, resulting in a low plasma bicarbonate and an elevated plasma chloride concentration.

   With improvements in the assays available for parathyroid hormone (PTH), such as whole molecule assays, this test now offers further diagnostic help in hypercalcaemia, when an inappropriate non-suppression of the hormone in hyperparathyroidism is usually observed. The serum PTH in our patient was 30 ng/l. If hyperparathyroidism is observed, then it is necessary to differentiate between primary, secondary or tertiary hyperparathyroidism, although this should be self-evident from the history. Furthermore, in cases of primary hyperparathyroidism, the multiple endocrine neoplasia (MEN) syndromes should be excluded. Assays for parathyroid hormone related peptide (PTH-RP) are also available and useful in some cases of malignant disease in which the syndrome of humoral hypercalcaemia is suspected. When trying to exclude malignant causes of hypercalcaemia, multiple myeloma should be excluded by performing serum and urine protein electrophoresis. Some textbooks allude to the steroid suppression test in which it is claimed that the hypercalcaemia of malignancy is reduced by hydrocortisone, unlike the hypercalcaemia due to excess PTH secretion. However, beware of false-positive and false-negative responses. Investigations are usually dictated by the clinical history and examination of the patient.

Drugs are a common cause of hypercalcaemia, notably thiazide diuretics, lithium and vitamin D. As our patient was not taking any medication, these can be excluded. The history obviously excluded immobilization as a cause of his hypercalcaemia, while the milk-alkali syndrome was unlikely, particularly in respect of a normal plasma bicarbonate concentration. Sarcoidosis and other granuloma conditions can also elicit hypercalcaemia as can thyrotoxicosis and Addison's disease. These can be excluded by appropriate investigations, which may include chest X-ray, plasma angiotensin-converting enzyme, thyroid function tests and the Synacthen test. Some causes of hypercalcaemia are given in *Table 8*.

3. Taking all that has been previously stated regarding investigations of hypercalcaemia and that fortuitiously this patient had a low urinary excretion of calcium in comparison to other causes of hypercalcaemia (which are often greater than 5 mmol per day), then the most likely diagnosis is familial hypocalciuric hypercalcaemia (FHH). This condition has also been named familial benign hypercalcaemia, which may be preferable as absolute hypocalciuria is not always present. The diagnosis is supported by the fact that this is an autosomal dominant condition and in our patient his family history seemed to suggest that his father had been investigated for a

Table 8 Some causes of hypercalcaemia

Primary (or tertiary) hyperparathyroidism
Malignant disease, multiple myeloma and multiple endocrine
neoplasia syndromes
Drugs
• Thiazides
• Milk-alkali syndrome
• Lithium
• Vitamin A or D excess
Granulomatous disease, e.g. sarcoidosis, tuberculosis
Endocrine
• Thyrotoxicosis
• Adrenal insufficiency
• Acromegaly
• Phaeochromocytoma
Immobilization
Familial hypocalciuric hypercalcaemia

'calcium problem'. Other family members should be screened for the condition. The subject is usually asymptomatic and the condition tends to take a benign course. It is important to distinguish FHH from primary hyperparathyroidism as removal of the parathyroid glands is contraindicated.

There has been some debate about which are the most useful investigations to diagnose this condition. A possible improvement in measuring the urinary calcium is to measure a fasting urinary calcium excretion index, that is to say the urine calcium concentration multiplied by the ratio of plasma to urine creatinine concentration. Plasma magnesium also tends to be elevated and can be a useful pointer. There have been suggestions that urinary excretion of hydroxyproline (a product of bone resorption) is normal in FHH, whereas this substance is elevated in primary hyperparathyroidism. Another suggested investigation is urinary phosphate excretion which tends to be increased in primary hyperparathyroidism compared to FHH. Alternatively, the phosphate excretion threshold can be measured. Confusion can result when measuring serum PTH as this can be normal or even elevated in FHH, probably due to a degree of parathyroid gland hyperplasia.

Case 13

A 59-year-old shop-keeper was referred to the general surgeons because of a recent change in bowel habit and the passage of blood per rectum. A barium enema had shown the presence of a colonic carcinoma and he was admitted for surgery to remove the tumour. Prior to admission, he had been healthy, was on no medication and did not smoke. Physical examination was unremarkable with no palpable abdominal masses or lymphadenopathy. A pre-operative determination of serum carcinoembryonic antigen (CEA) was 23 µg/l. He made a good postoperative recovery after his left colectomy, when it was also noticed that his liver showed no evidence of metastatic spread. However, histology showed a stage III tumour, which had invaded local lymph nodes. Before leaving hospital, a repeat serum CEA was 5 µg/l. He was followed-up regularly in the surgical out-patient clinic, but at 10 months post-operation his serum CEA was shown to be 16 µg/l.

Questions

1. What is the value of measuring serum CEA in this patient?
2. Explain the pattern of his serum CEA results.
3. Define what is meant by the sensitivity and specificity of a test.
4. For what tumours, is there merit in measuring CA 19–9, CA15–3 and CA–125?

Answers

1. Serum CEA is the term given to a family of glycoproteins originating from predominantly gastrointestinal epithelia. It has a role as a tumour marker for gastrointestinal malignancies, as well as some breast, ovarian and bronchial carcinomas. However, it can also be elevated in smokers, inflammatory bowel disease and pulmonary infections. In view of this nonspecificity, serum CEA has a limited role in the primary diagnosis of gastrointestinal carcinoma. However, with the patient as his own control, it does have a value, when sequential samples are taken, in monitoring tumour therapy and in the detection of tumour recurrence.

2. The pre-operative serum values of CEA of about 23 µg/l would be typical of a patient with a grade III gastrointestinal tumour. Apparent surgical removal of the tumour or decreasing tumour bulk resulted in the relatively normal serum CEA values of 5 µg/l. Unfortunately, the increase in serum CEA 10 months later suggests that the tumour had recurred.

3. It has been mentioned above that other conditions besides gastrointestinal malignancies can result in elevated serum CEA levels – thus limiting its use in the primary diagnosis of, or screening for, gut neoplasms. The ideal screening test should be both 100% specific for the condition in question and 100% sensitive, i.e. it should always detect individuals with the disease (no false negatives) but without turning up false positives (individuals without the disease). Specificity is defined as the incidence of true negative values in individuals without the disease. Sensitivity is defined as the incidence of true positive results in individuals with the disease. The sensitivity and specificity of a test also depend upon the prevalence of the disease in the population, and it is helpful to talk about the positive or negative predictive values of a test. The former is defined as the number of postive tests shown by subjects having the disease divided by the total number of tests that were positive. The latter is given by the number of negative tests shown by subjects not having the disease divided by the total number of negative tests.

4. These are all tumour markers, with the CA standing for carbohydrate antigen. CA 19–9 is related to some blood group compounds and has been shown to be elevated in certain gastrointestinal malignancies and also pancreatic carcinomas. CA 15–3 has been used as a marker for breast carcinoma and is in some way related to milk fat globulin. CA–125 is used in monitoring certain ovarian carcinomas.

Case 14

A 38-year-old window-cleaner was referred to the hospital lipid clinic having three months previously been discharged from hospital following an anterior myocardial infarction. It was noted at this time that the patient had a family history of premature coronary artery disease with his father having died at the age of 43 years from a myocardial infarction and his paternal uncle having died of the same at the age of 50 years. A serum cholesterol performed on admission to the coronary care unit had shown a concentration of 9.7 mmol/l. The patient smoked 20 cigarettes per day and drunk eight units of beer per week. He had been previously in good health apart from the myocardial infarction, having had no operations nor was he taking any medication. He had a common-law wife by whom he had two boys aged 10 and 8 years. On examination, he had a blood pressure of 130/72 and a body mass index of 26.7; examination was otherwise unremarkable except for bilateral tendon xanthomata upon the dorsum of his hands and Achilles tendons. He also had bilateral senile arcus. Resting ECG showed ischaemic changes. Fasting blood lipids revealed a serum cholesterol of 10.5 mmol/l, triglycerides of 1.6 mmol/l and high-density lipoprotein (HDL)-cholesterol of 1.0 mmol/l.

Questions

1. What is the most likely diagnosis?
2. What further biochemical investigations may be of relevance?
3. What other biochemical conditions can result in tendon xanthomata?
4. What was the calculated serum low-density lipoprotein LDL-cholesterol in this patient when he attended the lipid clinic?

Answers

1. The diagnosis is familial hypercholesterolaemia (FH). This condition is inherited as an autosomal dominant disorder. The inheritance of one mutant gene that encodes for the LDL-receptor affects about 1 in every 500 people, and results in impaired LDL-catabolism and hypercholesterolaemia. At least four types of mutation of the LDL-receptor have been described, resulting in either reduced synthesis, failure of transport of the synthesized receptor to the Golgi complex within the cell, defective LDL-binding or inadequate expression of the LDL-receptor at the cell surface.

Classically, these patients manifest severe hypercholesterolaemia, with a relatively normal serum triglyceride concentration and xanthomata which can affect the back of the hands, elbows, Achilles tendons or the insertion of the pateller tendon insertion into the pretibial tuberosity. This patient clearly illustrates some of these hyperlipidaemia stigmata and he also has premature cardiovascular disease which is frequent in this disorder.

Using the Frederickson's classification based upon serum lipoprotein electrophoresis, this condition has also been termed familial type II hyperlipoproteinaemia. Recently, it has been shown that in FH there is an increased amount of lipoprotein(a) which presumably contributes to the increased cardiovascular disease seen in these patients.

Homozygous FH is a rare condition showing extremely elevated serum cholesterol and the presence of tendon and cutaneous xanthomata in childhood. Severe coronary artery disease is usual before the age of 30, with frequent atheromatous lesions involving the aortic root.

2. The diagnosis of FH is usually obvious from the severely elevated serum cholesterol and the presence of tendon xanthomata in the patient or first-degree relative. The diagnosis may not be so clear-cut in patients without the lipid stigmata. A functional assay of the LDL-receptors has recently been described using cultured lymphocytes, but this has not yet gained wide acceptance.

In unclear cases, it is also worthwhile excluding secondary causes of hypercholesterolaemia, which include obstructive liver disease, nephrotic syndrome and hypothyroidism. Thus liver function tests, renal function tests including serum urea, electrolytes, and albumin, as well as urinary protein and thyroid function tests are of value.

Other lipid disorders giving rise to an elevation in serum cholesterol with a comparatively normal serum triglyceride concentration are worth mentioning (*Table 9*). Polygenic hypercholesterolaemia is as the name suggests, a condition resulting in an elevated serum cholesterol due to both genetic and enviromental factors, such as diet. One of the implicated genes is the E4 allele; apolipoprotein E being important for the binding of the remnant lipoprotein particle to its receptor. Another condition is familial defective apoB100 which has been recently described using gene probes. Apolipoprotein B100 is important in the binding of the LDL particle to its receptor.

Table 9 Some causes of hypercholesterolaemia (with a near-normal serum triglyceride concentration)

Primary	*Secondary*
• Familial hypercholesterolaemia	• Hypothyroidism
• Polygenic hypercholesterolaemia	• Nephrotic syndrome
• Familial apoB100 defects	• Cholestasis
• Cholesterol ester storage disease	• Diabetes mellitus
• Familial hyperalphalipoproteinaemia	• Acute intermittent porphyria
(HDL-cholesterol elevated)	• Anorexia nervosa
	• Chlorinated hydrocarbons

3. Cerebrotendinous xanthomatosis is a rare familial sterol storage disorder. It is inherited as an autosomal recessive disease and results in the accumulation of cholestanol and cholesterol in the tissues. It is characterized by cerebeller ataxia, spinal cord paresis and dementia. The other biochemical condition that can result in xanthomata is sitosterolaemia, another autosomal recessive disorder of sterol storage. As well as xanthomata, these patients have an increased risk of premature atherosclerosis. Increased amounts of the plant sterols, sitosterol and campesterol, are found in certain tissues and the plasma. Consider also type III hyperlipidaemia.

4. Using the Friedewald equation, the derived serum LDL – cholesterol is equal to total cholesterol – HDL-cholesterol – triglyceride/2.2 when the answer is expressed as mmol/l. In this patient, the equation is valid as the serum triglyceride concentration is less than 5 mmol/l – the correct answer for LDL-cholesterol being 8.8 mmol/l.

Case 15

A 44-year-old office clerk had been urgently referred to the hospital hypertension clinic because of his blood pressure. He smoked 15 cigarettes per day and consumed eight units of lager per week. He was on no medication, apart from a calcium-antagonist that his general practitioner had prescribed for his hypertension. His previous health was excellent, with his only previous medical attendance due to a broken nose sustained in a sporting accident. He had initially presented to his general practitioner with headaches and occasional polyuria. In the clinic, his blood pressure was 160/110 standing and 158/104 lying down. Physical examination was otherwise unremarkable, apart from grade one hypertensive retinopathy.

Blood was taken in the clinic for laboratory analysis and the following results were obtained: sodium 145 mmol/l; potassium 2.9 mmol/l; bicarbonate 38 mmol/l; chloride 90 mmol/l; urea 6.8 mmol/l; creatinine 0.12 mmol/l; random venous plasma glucose 4.4 mmol/l.

He reattended the clinic one week later when a 24-hour urine test was performed. This produced a total volume of 2.8 l with a potassium excretion of 56 mmol/l, a normal 4-hydroxy-3-methoxy mandelic acid (HMMA) and normal urinary free cortisol. Subsequently, he was admitted as an in-patient for investigations for possible Conn's syndrome.

Questions

1. Why did this patient's doctors wonder about Conn's syndrome?
2. What investigations should be performed in this patient?

Answers

1. Conn's syndrome or primary hyperaldosteronism should be considered in a hypertensive individual who has hypokalaemia. This patient has a hypokalaemic metabolic alkalosis; note the elevated plasma bicarbonate. Four main types of primary hyperaldosteronism have been described. The commonest is due to an adrenal adenoma, the next most common is adrenal hyperplasia, followed by the rarer dexamethasone-suppressible form, and finally adrenal carcinoma. Overall, primary hyperaldosteronism accounts for about 1% of all cases of hypertension. Due to the action of excess aldosterone secretion, there is potassium loss from the kidneys, resulting in hypokalaemia. Aldosterone is also a sodium-retaining hormone; this results in an increase in both extracellular and plasma volumes and thus hypertension. Also note that this patient's plasma sodium is at the upper limit of normal and he

is clearly hypokalemic with an inappropriate urinary excretion of potassium. Some authors state that provided the patient is taking an adequate sodium intake of greater than 120 mmol/l per day and that they are not taking potassium-losing drugs, then a urinary potassium loss of greater than 30 mmol/day indicates a renal kaliuresis. This patient's symptoms of polyuria are of note and probably reflect a nephrogenic form of diabetes insipidus due to long-standing hypokalaemia. Other symptoms sometimes experienced by these patients include polydipsia, nocturia, muscle weakness and paraesthesiae.

2. Certainly hypokalaemia and inappropriate urinary loss of potassium are pointers to a mineralocorticoid excess. Some clinicians would even consider a plasma potassium of below 4.0 mmol/l indicative of hyperaldosteronism in the presence of hypertension. One therefore needs to have a high index of suspicion if this diagnosis is not to be missed. Remember that potassium-losing diuretics can result in hypokalaemia and thus should be ideally stopped for at least two weeks prior to testing. High sodium intake can sometimes uncover hypokalaemia in a previously normokalaemic subject.

A popular method for determining the diagnosis of primary hyperaldosteronism is to measure plasma aldosterone and also renin activity in the morning, after the patient has been supine for at least half an hour, and then to repeat these measurements after four hours' ambulation. High plasma concentrations of aldosterone and low renin activity indicate primary hyperaldosteronism. Additionally, if the plasma aldosterone concentration falls on standing, this is indicative of an adrenal adenoma as opposed to adrenal hyperplasia when a rise is more usual.

Another discriminatory test between these variants of primary hyperaldosteronism is the measurement of plasma 18-hydroxy corticosterone, which is said to be higher in adenomas. An alternative dynamic test is to infuse angiotensin II which causes a large rise in plasma aldosterone in hyperplasia, but little or no response in the presence of an adenoma. In equivocal cases, some authors advocate aldosterone-suppression tests, either by saline infusion or by giving fludrocortisone or the angiotensin-converting enzyme (ACE) inhibitor, captopril. Normal subjects or those with essential hypertension usually suppress their plasma aldosterone concentrations under these circumstances.

Scanning by computer tomography is of use in further distinguishing between an adrenal adenoma and bilateral hyperplasia, as can scintiscanning using 19-iodocholesterol or 6-iodo-methyl 19-norcholesterol. Adrenal venous catheterization and sampling for aldosterone via a femoral vein is also useful in discriminating between an adenoma and hyperplasia. Furthermore, a trial of dexamethasone can be of use in establishing the suppressible variety of primary hyperaldosteronism.

In passing, it is worth mentioning those syndromes of secondary hyperaldosteronism, in which an elevated plasma aldosterone is observed in association with an elevated plasma renin activity. There are many conditions resulting in secondary hyperaldosteronism, including:

- Increased renin production due to renovascular hypertension or renin-secreting tumours.
- Oedematous states, such as cirrhosis, congestive cardiac failure and nephrotic syndrome.
- Increased renal electrolyte loss, e.g. Bartter's syndrome or diuretic usage.
- Hypovolaemic states, as in vomiting and haemorrhage.

Remember also that large consumption of liquorice or carbenoxolone, which both have mineralocorticoid activity can mimick primary hyperaldosteronism. Cushing's syndrome can also present with hypertension and hypokalaemia, but this was considered unlikely in this patient because of the lack of Cushingoid features and the normal urinary free cortisol result. There is also a syndrome of pseudohyperaldosteronism (Liddle's syndrome) in which hypertension and hypokalaemia can co-exist but there is a low plasma aldosterone. This is thought to be a hereditary disorder due to a renal tubular defect.

Case 16

A 56-year-old printer was brought to casualty by his wife because he was in a stupor. Obtaining a medical history was difficult because of his drowsiness. However, he complained of blurred vision. His wife explained that he had been previously well and was not taking any medication. She also explained that he was a non-smoker but that he was 'partial to a drink', as home-brewing was his avid hobby. On physical examination, he smelt of alcohol, had slight epigastric tenderness and a blood pressure of 98/70. A number of emergency blood tests were sent to the laboratory and some of these results are shown: sodium 140 mmol/l; potassium 4.0 mmol/l; chloride 93 mmo/l; bicarbonate 7 mmol/l; random venous plasma glucose 3.8 mmol/l; urea 5.2 mmol/l; creatinine 0.12 mmol/l; plasma osmolality 330 mmol/kg; paracetamol and salicylate not detected; amylase 376 U/l; ethanol not detected.

Questions

1. What is this patient's plasma anion gap?
2. What is the plasma osmolality gap in this patient?
3. What is the acid/base disturbance present in this patient?
4. Give a differential diagnosis and other relevant biochemical investigations.

Answers

1. The plasma anion gap is 44 mmol/l in this patient. This is calculated by the following formula: sodium + potassium plasma concentrations – chloride and bicarbonate plasma concentrations. Normally this value or 'gap' comes to between 10-16 mmol/l. An increased anion gap suggests an increase in the plasma unmeasured anions, such as might occur with renal failure, ketoacidosis, high salicylate intake, lactic acidosis, or a large consumption of ethanol, methanol or ethylene glycol. In theory, an increased anion gap could also be due to a decrease in unmeasured cations, such as calcium or magnesium, although in practice this is very rare.
2. The osmolality gap is the difference between the measured plasma osmolality and calculated osmolality. The calculated plasma osmolality approximates to 2 (sodium + potassium plasma concentrations) + urea plasma concentration + glucose plasma concentration. In practice, this gap is about 5 mmol/kg and a negative gap infers an analytical error. However, this patient has an osmolality gap of about 33 mmol/kg. This suggests the presence of an unmeasured substance in the

plasma which has contributed to the measured osmolality determination. This could include ethanol, methanol, ethylene glycol or drugs.

3. This patient has a low plasma bicarbonate which in itself could be due to either a metabolic acidosis or a compensated respiratory alkalosis. However, the increased anion gap and the magnitude of the plasma bicarbonate concentration clearly point to the former. The blood gases of this patient later showed a pH of 7.20, $PaCO_2$ 25 mmHg, and PaO_2 98 mmHg. The low blood $PaCO_2$ is the result of respiratory compensation due to hyperventilation in an attempt to increase the blood's pH.

Reasons for a metabolic acidosis (*Table 10*) include those causes of an increased plasma anion gap mentioned above. Other causes of a metabolic acidosis, in which a normal anion gap can be observed, include those conditions leading to bicarbonate loss, such as from the gastrointestinal system, e.g. diarrhoea or fistulae, or from the kidneys, as in proximal renal tubular acidosis. If the kidneys are less able to excrete hydrogen ions, a metabolic acidosis can also occur, as in renal failure, distal renal tubular acidosis or deficiency of the mineralocorticoid hormones.

4. Taking the increased osmolality into consideration as well as the metabolic acidosis, one should consider lactic acidosis, ketoacidosis, or ingestion of large amounts of ethanol, methanol, ethylene glycol or drugs such as salicylate. Thus urine ketones should be measured and also plasma lactic acid. Plasma ethanol and salicylate were already measured and shown to be minimal. It later transpired that this patient had inadvertently swallowed about a pint of methanol which he had stored in the shed where he kept his home-brewed beer. One clue from his medical history was the blurred vision.

Table 10 Some causes of a metabolic acidosis

Acute or chronic renal failure
Lactic acidosis
Ketoacidosis diabetes mellitus
Overdose
• Ethanol
• Methanol
• Ethylene glycol
• Salicylate
Hyperchloraemic acidosis (normal anion gap acidosis)

Case 17

A 41-year-old taxidriver was seen in the endocrine clinic because of increased weight, muscle weakness and impotence. These symptoms had started about nine months previously and had been getting progressively worse. Prior to this, he had been in good health, with no history of operations, although he did admit to recently having an irritating non-productive cough and also having to get up at night twice to pass urine. He was a heavy smoker at 30 cigarettes per day, but only rarely consumed alcohol at weekends. He was taking no medication except for sleeping tablets. On physical examination, he looked slightly brown in appearance, his body mass index was 27.8 and his blood pressure was 168/100. His limbs appeared thin in proportion to the rest of his body and he manifested a proximal myopathy. In view of these findings, the endocrinologist suspected that Cushing's syndrome was a likely diagnosis and arranged for investigations. Some results of the routine biochemical screen were: sodium 146 mmol/l; potassium 3.4 mmol/l; urea 8.4 mmol/l; creatinine 0.12 mmol/l; random venous plasma glucose 12.0 mmol/l. Urinary free cortisol 1345 nmol/24 hours.

Plasma cortisol	9 am:	887 nmol/l
	midnight:	878 nmol/l
Plasma ACTH	9 am:	443 ng/l
	midnight:	398 ng/l

Low dose 2 mg dexamethasone suppression test

| 9 am before | plasma cortisol 896 nmol/l |
| 9 am after | plasma cortisol 805 nmol/l |

High dose 8 mg dexamethasone suppression test

9 am plasma cortisol after test 784 nmol/l

Questions

1. What is the diagnosis and suggest a possible explanation for these results?
2. What further investigations may be necessary in confirming the diagnosis?

Answers

1. The patient's history and physical findings, as well as the biochemical results, confirm that the patient has Cushing's syndrome almost certainly due to an ectopic ACTH source. Note the relatively short clinical history, the overt diabetes mellitus and hypokalaemia of this patient. Furthermore, there is an elevated 24-hour urinary free cortisol, loss of cortisol diurnal variation (midnight plasma cortisol is normally less than 220 nmol/l), absence of a significant response to both low-dose and high-dose dexamethasone suppression and high plasma ACTH concentrations. All these findings strongly suggest an ectopic ACTH source as the reason for his Cushing's syndrome. He also showed pigmentation which fits with an elevated ACTH.

   Adrenal carcinoma or adenoma can be reasonably excluded because although they too could result in a failure of both low-dose and high-dose dexamethasone to suppress plasma cortisol, the plasma ACTH concentration would be expected to be low or undetectable. Also, these patients tend to show signs of virilism due to excess adrenal androgen production. The most likely source of diagnostic confusion with an ectopic ACTH source is pituitary dependent Cushing's disease. Here hypokalaemia is rare and most patients with pituitary dependent Cushing's disease show 50% or more suppression of basal plasma cortisol levels in response to the high-dose dexamethasone test. It would also be unusual for plasma ACTH concentrations to be as high as those found in this patient if there was pituitary-dependent Cushing's disease.

   A chest X-ray later showed that this man had a bronchial tumour which on biopsy proved to be an oat-cell carcinoma which was secreting ACTH. The other lung tumour that is well decribed as releasing ACTH is a bronchial carcinoid tumour.

2. The diagnosis of Cushing's syndrome in this patient is relatively clear-cut and should not cause too much confusion. Sometimes screening tests can be equivocal, particularly in obese patients, those with depression or in those with high ethanol intake (alcoholic pseudo-Cushing's syndrome). In some of these circumstances, an insulin tolerance test is useful. In Cushing's syndrome, high plasma cortisol suppresses the hypoglycaemic response, whereas in obesity or depression hypoglycaemia should evoke a rise in plasma cortisol by more than 220 nmol/l.

Some authors advocate the metyrapone test (metyrapone inhibits the 11-hydroxylase step in the glucocorticoid pathway) as a useful diagnostic test in Cushing's syndrome. Plasma 11-deoxycortisol is assayed; while patients with a primary adrenal pathology show little or no response, patients with pituitary-dependent Cushing's disease show an exaggerated response of both basal plasma ACTH and 11-deoxycortisol. However, so do some patients with an ectopic ACTH source. There has been recent interest in the corticotrophin releasing hormone test (CRH test). This can show an excessive response of ACTH in pituitary Cushing's disease, but an absence of ACTH response in an ectopic source.

Once a diagnosis of Cushing's syndrome has been made, the cause should be elucidated. Imaging techniques, such as computerized tomography scanning, are useful in searching for adrenal or pituitary pathology. Venous catheter studies can help localize ectopic ACTH sources in for example, the mediastinum, while petrosal sinus and jugular sampling may localize a pituitary source. In the event of a pituitary dependent ACTH source, an assessment of other pituitary hormones is usually warranted.

Case 18

A 21-year-old secretary was admitted to casualty with increasing breathlessness. She had been a known sufferer of asthma since a child, for which she regularly used a salbutamol inhaler. Over the last couple of days, she had noticed an increase in breathlessness associated with wheezing and she had developed a productive cough with green sputum. She was a non-smoker and her only other medication was the contraceptive pill. On examination she was tachypnoeic and had extensive wheezes throughout her chest, but was not cyanosed. Chest X-ray showed hyperinflated lungs and signs of a recent chest infection. Blood was taken for blood gases on admission and showed pH 7.40, PaO_2 of 88 mmHg and a $PaCO_2$ of 36 mmHg. She was commenced on intravenous hydrocortisone and antibiotics, and was given a salbutamol nebulizer and oxygen to inhale via a venti-mask before being sent to the medical ward. In the morning, the blood gases were repeated and blood was also sent for routine biochemistry. The results of the former were: sodium 144 mmol/l; potassium 3.0 mmol/l; urea 6.5 mmol/l; creatinine 0.10 mmol/l. The blood gas results showed pH 7.42, PaO_2 104 mmHg and $PaCO_2$ 38 mmHg. Clinically, the patient felt much better and her breathlessness had abated, with improvement in her peak-flow recording.

Questions

1. Why was the patient hypokalaemic?
2. What is the merit in measuring urinary potassium excretion in hypokalaemic patients?
3. Comment upon her initial blood gas result in relation to the severity of her asthmatic attack.

Answers

1. The hypokalaemia is almost certainly the result of the salbutamol administration. Beta-adrenergic agonists are known to result in a shift of potassium from the extracellular space to within the cells. Indeed, such drugs have been used to treat some cases of hyperkalaemia. A similar extracellular-to-intracellular shift is seen with insulin treatment, barium intoxication and following the treatment of pernicious anaemia with vitamin B_{12}. One should be vigilant in patients with asthma and taking beta-adrenergic agonists in case they develop hypokalaemia. Intracellular shifts of potassium resulting in hypokalaemia also occur in familial hypokalaemic periodic paralysis and hypothermia.
2. The urinary potassium would be expected to be low, i.e. below 10 mmol/l, in this patient. Other causes of hypokalemia resulting in a low urinary potassium include states giving rise to impaired potassium intake such as alcoholism, anorexia nervosa, geophagia and inadequate intravenous or parenteral therapy (*Table 11*). Furthermore, this would also be the case with gastrointestinal loss of potassium as might occur with fistulae, diarrhoea and villous adenoma of the rectum or colon. Conversely, a raised urinary potassium excretion, e.g. greater than 10 mmol/l in the presence of hypokalaemia, can be due

to a metabolic alkalosis (such as is seen with severe vomiting), diuretic therapy using either loop diuretics or thiazides, or the use of poorly reabsorbable anionic drugs, such as penicillin, and can also occur in association with hypomagnesaemia. Other causes of hypokalaemia associated with increased urinary potassium loss include renal disease affecting the renal tubules, e.g. post-urinary obstruction, Fanconi's syndrome, renal tubular acidosis (type 1 or 2) and in the transplanted kidney. Syndromes resulting in increased mineralocorticoid activity, such as primary and secondary hyperaldosteronism, Cushing's syndrome and the use of steroids, liquorice or carbenoxolone can also lead to hypokalaemia with increased urinary potassium loss. It should therefore be apparent that urinary determination of potassium can be a useful investigation in cases of hypokalaemia.

3. The initial blood gases of this patient suggest that her asthmatic attack was not *in extremis*. Fortunately, her $PaCO_2$ did not become elevated, i.e she did not become hypercapnic. In many cases of asthma, the $PaCO_2$ is low as a result of hyperventilation. A raised blood gas $PaCO_2$ and the development of a respiratory acidosis would suggest a patient is severely ill and may need mechanical ventilation. In patients with hypercapnia remember also that uncontrolled oxygen therapy can result in loss of their hypoxic drive and thus lead to further carbon dioxide retention.

Table 11 Some causes of hypokalaemia

Decreased intake	Poor dietary intake or inappropriate intravenous replacement
Redistribution	Alkalaemia
	Insulin
	Beta-adrenergic drugs or activity
	Hypokalaemic periodic paralysis
	Treatment of anaemias
	Hypothermia
Renal loss	Potassium-losing diuretics
	Fanconi's syndrome
	Mineralocorticoid excess syndromes
	Tubular damage
Gastrointestinal loss	Fistulae
	Diarrhoea
Hypomagnesaemia.	

Case 19

An 18-year-old unemployed male was brought to casualty because of a motorcycle accident in which he received a head injury. On admission, he was unconscious and was taken to intensive care for mechanical ventilation. In addition to his head injury, he had a fractured left femur and right clavicle. He regained consciousness within 12 hours and was transferred to the orthopaedic ward after a few days. The only drugs that he was taking at this time were analgesics and he was then able to eat and drink normally. It was noticed from the fluid-balance charts that the patient was passing large volumes of urine and he complained of thirst. A timed urine collection was made and was found to be 5.1 litres in 24 hours with an osmolality of 106 mmol/kg. Blood tests showed: sodium 144 mmol/l; potassium 4.5 mmol/l; urea 7.5 mmol/l; creatinine 0.12 mmol/l; random venous plasma glucose 4.1 mmol/l; calcium 2.31 mmol/l; phosphate 0.88 mmol/l; albumin 41 g/l.

Questions

1. What is the most likely explanation for the polyuria?
2. Discuss other causes of polyuria that can occur.
3. What investigations could be performed to confirm the diagnosis in this patient?

Answers

1. Polyuria is usually defined as the passage of more than 3 litres of urine per day. The patient probably has cranial diabetes insipidus as a result of his head injury. Vasopressin or antidiuretic hormone (ADH) is a peptide hormone released from the posterior pituitary. One of its actions is to increase water reabsorption by the renal tubules.
2. There are a number of causes of polyuria. It is first of all useful to always confirm suspected polyuria by a timed urine collection. Some workers have divided polyuria into either solute or water diuresis upon the basis of urine osmolality determinations, using an osmolality of greater than 300 mmol/kg to define the former and less than about 200 mmol/kg to define

the latter. The water diuresis group includes those conditions giving rise to diabetes insipidus and also individuals with a high water intake.

The diabetes insipidus group itself can be divided into cranial or nephrogenic forms. In the cranial variety, there is an impairment of ADH secretion due to damage to the hypothalamus or posterior pituitary, as may be seen after a head injury, cerebral tumours, cranial surgery, granulomas, infections and autoimmune disease, in which there is destruction of the hypothalamic nuclei that produce ADH. There is also the DIDMOAD syndrome, in which type 1 diabetes mellitus is associated with deafness and optic atrophy. In nephrogenic diabetes insipidus, the renal tubules lack the ability to respond to ADH. This can either be the result of an inherited sex-linked disorder or of acquired forms of renal disease, including hypercalcaemia, hypokalaemia and amyloidosis. Drugs can also be implicated, such as lithium.

Psychogenic or compulsive fluid drinkers can mimick diabetes insipidus and these individuals can consume vast amounts of water leading to polyuria. Remember also that chronic renal failure can result in polyuria, as can pyelonephritis and renal transplantation.

The solute group of polyuria includes diabetes mellitus, diuretic therapy, salt losing nephropathies, hypercatabolic states, parenteral nutrition and the administration of mannitol.

3. Having established whether the polyuria is a water or solute diuresis and having excluded the latter, a water deprivation test is frequently used to establish a diagnosis of diabetes insipidus, either due to a cranial source or the nephrogenic variety. A useful screening test is to determine the osmolality of an early morning urine sample; if this exceeds about 800 mmol/kg, this suggests the absence of diabetes insipidus. Normally, plasma osmolality is tightly regulated to between 280-290 mmol/kg. In diabetes insipidus, the plasma osmolality can exceed 295 mmol/kg if dehydration has taken place, i.e. if the water intake can not match the urinary and insensible losses.

Conversely, in primary or pyschogenic polydipsia, a low plasma osmolality of less than 274 mmol/kg may be seen. In the eight-hour fluid-deprivation test, careful patient monitoring is mandatory to ensure that the plasma osmolality does not exceed about 300 mmol/kg nor the patient lose more than 3% of their total body weight. In normal individuals during the test, an increase in urine osmolality to at least twice that of the plasma osmolality occurs, but the plasma osmolality barely rises. Furthermore, in normal subjects, the urine can be maximally concentrated during dehydration to about 1000 mmol/kg. However, the converse is true, in diabetes insipidus, with a rise in plasma osmolality but an impaired response of the urine concentration. Serial urine osmolalities are performed hourly and, when the results do not differ by more than 30 mmol/kg, vasopressin is administered. In the case of nephrogenic diabetes insipidus, there is no response to the vasopressin, i.e. there is no significant increase in urine osmolality because of tubular unresponsiveness to ADH, whereas in cranial diabetes insipidus the urine osmolality reaches 800 mmol/kg. Partial forms of both cranial and nephrogenic diabetes insipidus also exist. In pychogenic polydipsia, water deprivation causes urine osmolality to rise as normal with increasing plasma osmolality, although sometimes a prolonged water deprivation test may be necessary to highlight this.

Case 20

A 41-year-old man was referred to the medical outpatients' department because he was behaving uncharacteristically and was showing difficulty getting up out of a chair. He was educationally subnormal and had lived in a residential home since childhood. It was thought that he had experienced birth trauma and asphyxia. This resulted in brain damage which had caused him to become epileptic. During his childhood, he had been prescribed phenytoin which he still took in a daily dose of 300 mg. Unfortunately he spoke few words. However, physical examination revealed a blood pressure of 114/72 with little else of note, apart from an obvious weakness of the muscles affecting his pelvic girdle which was not associated with any bony pain. The clinician felt the diagnosis was clearcut and took biochemical and haematological blood tests which showed the following results: bilirubin 3 μmol/l; alkaline phosphatase 546 U/l; alanine transaminase 45 U/l; gamma-glutamyl transferase 232 U/l; albumin 36 g/l;

calcium 1.78 mmol/l; phosphate 0.66 mmol/l; phenytoin 30 mg/l; haemoglobin 12 g/dl; white cells 6.9 × 10⁹/l; platelets 256 × 10⁹/l.

Questions

1. What is the corrected plasma calcium?
2. Suggest the most likely diagnosis and what investigations would help to confirm this?
3. What other conditions can lead to a similar plasma calcium concentration?
4. The clinician was surprised at the serum phenytoin concentration. It later transpired that the patient had taken his dose just prior to his out-patient appointment. Comment upon the drug plasma levels.

Answers

1. The corrected calcium is 1.86 mmol/l. This is based on the formula: measured plasma calcium concentration + 0.02 × (40 − measured plasma albumin concentration g/l).
2. The most likely diagnosis is osteomalacia. This could be confirmed, as in this patient, by the characteristic X-ray changes and isotopic bone scan. If considered necessary, a bone biopsy would depict a deficit in the mineralization of osteoid. Note the hypocalcaemia, hypophosphataemia, and the elevated plasma alkaline phosphatase in this patient. Regarding the aetiology, it is probable that this is due to chronic use of the anticonvulsant phenytoin, although dietary factors can not be ruled out in this patient. It has been suggested that phenytoin is a powerful enzyme inducer, which probably also explains the elevated plasma gamma-glutamyl-transferase activity, and that this results in the metabolism of vitamin D into inactive metabolites. Although low plasma concentrations of 25-hydroxycholecalciferol have been described in such cases, there have also been surprising reports of normal plasma concentrations of 1,25 dihydroxy-cholecalciferol. Thus, it is likely that the osteomalacia is also partly related to nutritional factors and the relative lack of sunlight as a result of institutional life.

Other causes of osteomalacia include severe hypophos-phataemia, vitamin D deficiency due to malabsorption states, bone toxins including aluminium and fluoride, vitamin-D-dependent rickets and chronic renal failure.

3. When faced with a case of hypocalcaemia, one should first of all check the albumin-corrected calcium and exclude hypoalbuminaemic states. We have already discussed decreased calcium intake, whether the result of poor intake (either orally or parenterally) or of impaired vitamin D activity. Chronic renal failure is a common cause of hypocalcaemia in hospital patients, as is acute pancreatitis in which calcium is sequestered in extraskeletal tissues. Hypoparathyroidism and pseudohypoparathyroidism can also result in hypocalcaemia. A serum parathyroid hormone (PTH) determination is of value being undetectable or low in the case of the former, and abnormally elevated in the latter, as a result of a PTH-receptor binding defect. Drug causes of hypocalcaemia should not be forgotten and include glucocorticoids, calcitonin, frusemide, mithramycin and phosphate.

Hypocalcaemia can also be due to rarer conditions, including hypomagnesaemia, the so-called 'hungry bone syndrome' seen post-parathyroidectomy and ethylene glycol or colchicine poisoning, as well as following massive blood transfusion. In the latter case, calcium chelation by anticoagulant can reduce plasma ionized calcium concentration despite normal total plasma calcium concentrations. Ionized plasma calcium can also be low as a result of hyperventilation when tetany can be observed. *Table 12* lists some causes of hypocalaemia.

4. The therapeutic plasma range for phenytoin is about 10–20 mg/l and there is great individual variability in therapeutic response among patients. The phenytoin levels reported in this patient were elevated but this was simply because the blood sample was taken too close after ingestion of the drug

Table 12 Some causes of hypocalcaemia

Chronic renal failure
Poor intake of calcium or vitamin D deficiencies
Hypoparathyroidism and pseudohypoparathyroidism
Drugs, e.g. calcitonin, diphosphonates, loop diuretics, anticonvulsants
Ethylene glycol poisoning or fluoride toxicity
Acute pancreatitis
Intravenous magnesium or phosphate in excess
Neonatal varieties.

rather than at pre-dose. Phenytoin displays non-linear or Michaelis-Menten kinetics and thus small incremental changes in drug dose can lead to large changes in plasma levels of the drug. Toxic effects of phenytoin include paradoxical fitting, cerebellar syndrome, folate deficiency, inhibition of antidiuretic hormone release, gum hyperplasia and lymphadenopathy.

Case 21

A 61-year-old retired railway worker attended the cardiology clinic because of cardiac failure and an irregular heart beat. He had been put onto a thiazide diuretic, an angiotensin-converting enzyme inhibitor, and amiodarone. He had felt much better in terms of his breathlessness and orthopnoea since attending the clinic. He had stopped smoking three months previously and only consumed one pint of lager at weekends. Physical examination showed a blood pressure of 126/78, a regular pulse of 62 beats/min and nothing else of note except slightly oedematous ankles. He had no tremor and his eyes were normal. Thyroid function tests were sent to the laboratory and the following results were returned to the clinic: TSH 2.1 mU/l; fT4 27.3 pmol/l; fT3 6.2 pmol/l.

Questions

1. Why were thyroid function tests sent to the laboratory?
2. Give a possible explanation for the thyroid function results.
3. What are other causes of euthyroid hyperthyroxinaemia?

Answers

1. Amiodarone is a Class III antiarrhythmic drug and is an iodinated benzofuran derivative. However, approximately 40% of its weight is iodine. By inhibiting the deiodination of T4, this drug impairs the conversion of T4 to T3. There is also

evidence that amiodarone is a competitive inhibitor of T3 receptors and may also in some cases reduce TSH production in the pituitary gland. One of its actions is to evoke a state of hypothyroidism within the cardiac muscle. In view of these diverse actions upon thyroid status, amiodarone therapy can cause alterations in thyroid function and result in either hypothyroidism or conversely hyperthyroidism. For these reasons, patients starting amiodarone should have thyroid function tests performed at baseline and at about six-monthly intervals thereafter. Some have proposed that serum TSH is the best guide to thyroid function in these cases as a normal TSH concentration implies a euthyroid state. Others have suggested that, if there is a suspicion of thyroid dysfunction, then a thyrotrophin-releasing hormone (TRH) stimulation test is useful.

2. This patient shows an elevated fT4, but a normal TSH and a low normal fT3. He was clinically euthyroid which is supported by his TSH result. The most likely explanation for these findings is that the peripheral conversion of T4 to T3 is impaired by the amiodarone. Primary hyperthyroidism would be indicated if the TSH was suppressed and the fT4 and/or fT3 concentration was elevated, conversely hypothyroidism would be suggested by a raised TSH concentration and low thyroid hormones. This patient displays the condition of euthyroid hyperthyroxinaemia, i.e. raised plasma thyroxine (fT4 in this case) in a euthyroid patient.

3. Other causes that have been described for euthyroid hyperthyroxinaemia include other drugs, such as iodine-containing contrast media and the beta-blocker propranolol, which also impairs peripheral conversion of thyroxine (T4) to T3. Sometimes the phenomenon is seen in patients on thyroxine medication and a transient hyperthyroxinaemia has been described in various non-thyroid illnesses. An individual can also have an elevated plasma T4 concentration due to a degree of peripheral resistance of the tissues to thyroxine.

Another condition in which euthyroid hyperthyroxinaemia is displayed is when there is an abnormality of thyroid-hormone-binding proteins. If these proteins are present in excess amounts, or have an enhanced affinity for thyroxine, then elevated plasma concentrations of the hormone will be apparent. This will also depend to some extent upon the assay method to determine plasma thyroxine concentrations. The older methods measured total hormone levels but there is now a tendency to use free hormone assays, i.e. they quantitate the non-bound hormone or supposedly active form of the hormone. However, depending upon the methodology, these free hormone assays (usually the analogue methods rather than equilibrium dialysis) can sometimes still show elevated free hormone concentrations in the presence of abnormal or excess plasma-binding-proteins. Thyroid-binding globulin (TBG) is one of the principal thyroid-binding proteins in plasma; and sometimes plasma TBG can be found in excess resulting in euthyroid hyperthyroxinaemia. Albumin and also pre-albumin can bind thyroxine in plasma; there are inherited molecular variants that show increased affinity for thyroxine and thus also result in a euthyroid hyper-thyroxinaemic state. Some individuals can have circulating antibodies that bind to thyroxine, and a spuriously elevated hormone concentration can similarly occur in some thyroid hormone assays.

Case 22

A 10-year-old boy was admitted by the surgical team because of an acute onset of abdominal pain. The pain was located mainly in his epigastric region and radiated through to his back. This was associated with nausea. From his past medical history, it transpired that he had suffered from an attack one year previously. Otherwise he was a healthy boy of average height and weight for his age. There was nothing of note in the family history. On examination his blood pressure was 90/60 and he was markedly tender in his epigastric region. He also had hepato-splenomegaly. Rectal examination was normal. The house-surgeon noticed 'acne'-like spots on his thighs and buttocks, but otherwise nothing else of remark. A provisional diagnosis of acute pancreatitis was made and emergency blood was taken for electrolytes and urea, glucose and amylase. The following results were obtained: sodium 128 mmol/l; potassium 3.7 mmol/l; urea 7.8 mmol/l; random venous plasma glucose 4.3 mmol/l; amylase was reported as not detected. The sample was also reported as being lipaemic.

Questions

1. Explain the biochemical findings.
2. What is the most likely diagnosis?
3. Discuss further investigations that are necessary to establish the diagnosis.

Answers

1. The presence of hyponatraemia in a lipaemic sample should alert the clinician and the laboratory to the phenomenon of pseudohyponatraemia. A quick method of determining this is to measure the plasma osmolality and to also calculate the plasma osmolality from the following approximation; plasma calculated osmolality equals 2(sodium + potassium plasma concentration) + urea plasma concentration + glucose plasma concentration. The measured and calculated plasma osmolalities should be approximately similar, but if the measured osmolality greatly exceeds the calculated value and if hyponatraemia and lipaemia are present, then pseudohyponatraemia is suggested. The reason for this phenomenon is that despite the sodium ions being present only in the plasma water space, the results are expressed and measured in terms of total plasma volume by certain instruments, such as indirect ion-selective electrodes or flame-emission spectroscopy. If the water space of the plasma is reduced by the occupation of high amounts of lipids or protein (as in multiple myeloma), then a factitiously low plasma sodium concentration will result.

   The other point of remark is the undetected amylase activity; one should also be aware that enzyme activities can be difficult to measure in lipaemic samples. If pancreatitis is suspected in such cases, then either the plasma lipids should be separated by centrifugation or filtration and then amylase determined, or urinary amylase should be assayed. Sometimes, the plasma sample can be diluted with saline and then the enzyme assay repeated.

2. Taking the clinical findings and the lipaemic sample into consideration, a diagnosis of acute pancreatitis secondary to hypertriglyceridaemia should be seriously considered. Further investigations showed serum triglycerides of 78.9 mmol/l and cholesterol of 7.6 mmol/l. A serum sample stored at 4°C overnight in a fridge revealed a top layer of 'cream'

showing chylomicrons. Serum lipoprotein electrophoresis confirmed a Fredrickson's type 1 or chylomicronaemic hyperlipidaemia. This is the result of a defect in the activity of the enzyme lipoprotein lipase.

The most usual form of this disorder is familial lipoprotein lipase deficiency, an autosomal recessive disorder affecting about one in every one million people. The boy's age and his presentation with pancreatitis are typical and the condition is characterized by grossly elevated serum triglycerides due to the accumulation of uncleared chylomicron particles. Eruptive xanthomata occur classically on the thigh and buttock – hence the description of 'acne' by the house-surgeon – along with hepatosplenomegaly and lipaemia retinalis. Other variants of the chylomicron syndrome include circulating inhibitors of lipoprotein lipase and deficiency of its physiological activator, apolipoprotein CII.

Other conditions which can sometimes be confused with the syndrome because hypertriglyceridaemia is observed is familial hypertriglyceridaemia showing either the type IV or type V Frederickson's phenotype. In the former, the elevated serum triglyceride is due largely to an increase in the very-low-density lipoprotein (VLDL) particles, while in the latter a combination of elevated VLDL and chylomicrons are observed. Secondary causes of hypertriglyceridaemia include obesity, high ethanol consumption, diabetes mellitus, glycogen storage disease and progressive partial lipodystrophy. Certain drugs can aggravate hypertriglyceridaemia, such as oestrogens, glucocorticoids and thiazides. *Table 13* gives some causes of a predominant hypertriglyceridaemia.

Table 13 Some causes of a predominant hypertriglyceridaemia

Primary	Secondary
Chylomicron syndrome	Obesity
• Familial lipoprotein lipase deficiency	Ethanol
	Diabetes mellitus
• Inhibitor of lipoprotein lipase	Chronic renal failure
• ApoC II deficiency	Glucocorticoids
Familial hypertriglyceridaemia	Thiazides
• Type IV	Glycogen-storage disease
• Type V	Progressive partial lipodystrophy
Hepatic lipase deficiency	

3. To confirm the diagnosis of familial lipoprotein lipase deficiency plasma lipoprotein lipase can be assayed after the intravenous administration of heparin, which releases the enzyme from endothelial sites. The assay is complicated in that other plasma lipases (due to hepatic lipase and phospholipase for example) contribute to the overall plasma lipase activity. Inhibition of lipoprotein lipase can be performed either using protamine, high saline concentrations or specific antibodies and its overall activity calculated by subtraction. If apo-CII deficiency is suspected then the serum concentration of this activator can be assayed and if an inhibitor of lipoprotein lipase is considered then adipose tissue lipoprotein lipase can be measured which should be normal or high in activity in comparison to plasma levels which are reduced. Alternatively, one can try diluting out the inhibitor, in vitro, with the plasma from a normal individual. Useful supportive information of a lipoprotein lipase abnormality can be gleaned from the low fat test when the patient is subjected to a low fat diet (usually less than 10 g of daily fat) when there should be a reduction in the formation of chylomicrons. As the condition is inherited other family members should be investigated.

Case 23

A 31-year-old house-wife had been referred to the endocrine clinic because of tiredness, weakness and absent periods. She had been getting progressively more lethargic over the past 11 months and had noticed that, over a similar time, her periods were becoming erratic and now had finally ceased. On direct questioning she admitted losing 3 kg in weight recently and to feeling dizzy when she got up from sitting. When asked, she also stated that she had noticed a couple of small white areas of skin appearing on her left arm. She was not on any medication and had previously been in good health, having had no operations or serious illnesses. She was a non-smoker and only rarely consumed alcohol. Her mother apparently had a problem with her thyroid gland and took tablets for this. Her sister had a muscle disease and anaemia.

Physical examination showed blood pressure of 102/70 with a marked postural drop. The doctor also noticed areas of pigmentation within her mouth and also areas of vitiligo upon her arms. He also noticed slow relaxing ankle jerks. Several blood tests were requested and the results of some of the chemistry tests are shown here: sodium 130 mmol/l; potassium 5.7 mmol/l; urea 7.5 mmol/l; creatinine 0.12 mmol/l; calcium 2.68 mmol/l; phosphate 0.98 mmol/l; albumin 41 g/l; random venous plasma glucose 12.4 mmol/l; TSH 17.2 mU/l; fT4 4.6 pmol/l; LH 36 U/l; FSH 54 U/l; prolactin 245 mU/l; random morning cortisol 79 nmol/l.

Questions

1. Comment upon these biochemical findings and suggest a likely diagnosis.
2. What further investigations should be performed to assess her adrenal function?
3. What other disorders is this condition associated with?

Answers

1. The patient clearly has primary hypothyroidism, as judged by an elevated serum TSH and low fT4. This would also fit with the slow relaxing ankle jerks. The elevated gonadotrophins point to a primary ovarian abnormality, which would partly account for her menstrual problems. The low random cortisol concentration also suggests adrenal insufficiency (Addison's disease) which would be in keeping with some of her symptoms – the postural drop in blood pressure and her buccal pigmentation (due to elevated ACTH). Plasma cortisol shows diurnal variation with the highest levels normally in the morning, usually between 180–720 nmol/l. The electrolyte results showing hyponatraemia and hyperkalaemia substantiate this. Interestingly, plasma calcium can also be moderately elevated in adrenal insufficiency and sometimes the plasma urea is also found to be elevated. Note also that the plasma glucose concentration is high and fulfills the WHO criteria of diabetes mellitus. Thus, the patient has presented with multiple endocrine gland failure. This would be entirely consistent with type II polyendocrine autoimmune disease, also known as Schmidt's disease.

2. The low morning plasma cortisol and the biochemical and clinical features of this patient clearly point to adrenal insufficiency. If done at this time, a simultaneous plasma ACTH determination would be expected to be elevated in Addison's disease. In equivocal cases, the short Synacthen test can be performed. If the plasma cortisol rises by more than 200 nmol/l to a concentration greater than 600 nmol/l, then Addison's disease is usually excluded. Note in the normal short Synacthen response, the 30-minute cortisol sample is greater than the 60-minute sample. Also note that the prolonged Synacthen test is primarily used to investigate adrenal insufficiency secondary to pituitary or hypothalamic disease or patients on steroid treatment. Serum autoantibody determination would also be of value to detect the presence of adrenal, thyroid, ovarian and pancreatic islet cell antibodies.

3. Schmidt's syndrome can be associated with alopecia, pernicious anaemia, myasthenia gravis (note that her sister had a 'muscle disease' and anaemia) and vitiligo. These conditions should also be looked for in such patients. There is also a familial tendency, with some authors suggesting an autosomal recessive inheritance. This condition should not be confused with the type 1 polyendocrine autoimmune syndrome in which features of adrenal insufficiency, hypoparathyroidism and candidiasis infections are observed.

Case 24

A 22-year-old shopworker was referred to the dermatology clinic because of an acute onset of photosensitivity. She complained that she had suffered two previous attacks in the preceding summer but her current episode was the worst of all. Her past medical history was unremarkable except that she had a pregnancy termination five years previously. She smoked five cigarettes per day and consumed four units of alcohol per week. Her only medication was the oral contraceptive pill. She thought her mother also suffered from a similar skin rash particularly in summer months.

Examination was also unremarkable, with a blood pressure of 105/72. However, there were erythematous and oedematous skin lesions on the sunexposed areas of her face and arms. There was no skin scarring and the skin showed no thickening. The consultant dermatologist decided that the skin lesions were typical of protoporphyria. Urine, faeces and blood were sent to the clinical chemistry laboratory for analysis, and the following results were obtained (with normal ranges in parentheses):

- Urine porphobilinogen (PBG), 5 μmol/l (0–10)
- Urine total porphyrins, 50 nmol/l (20–330)
- Faecal total porphyrins, 380 nmol/g dry weight (10–210)
- Erythrocyte porphyrins, 148 μmol/l (0.5–2).

Fluorescence emission spectra, using an excitation wavelength of 405 nm, of both an ethanol extract from whole blood and also a plasma sample showed large fluorescence peaks at 632 nm. Other results included: bilirubin 14 μmol/l, alanine transaminase 23 U/l; alkaline phosphatase 76 U/l.

Questions

1. Do these results support the diagnosis of protoporphyria?
2. What would the same biochemical tests show in porphyria cutanea tarda?
3. What is the biochemical defect in protoporphyria?
4. How can lead toxicity cause changes in erythrocyte porphyrins?

Answers

1. These findings strongly support the diagnosis of protoporphyria. Indeed, the skin lesions are typical and to an experienced dermatologist should point to a diagnosis of protoporphyria. However, all the porphyrias, except for acute intermittent porphyria and PBG-synthase deficiency, can result in skin manifestations. With protoporphyria excluded, the other porphyrias tend to result in subepidermal bullae, increased skin fragility and areas of pigmentation.

   The elevated erythrocyte porphyrins suggest an erythrocyte porphyria. The two common forms are protoporphyria and congenital erythropoietic porphyria (CEP). The latter can show elevated urinary porphyrins of the uroporphyrin I and copro-porphyrin I types and also a plasma fluorescence peak at 615 nm. The defect in CEP is a deficiency of the enzyme uropor-phyrinogen III synthase and is inherited as an autosomal reces-sive condition. In addition, CEP is a rare disorder affecting about 1 in a million people. The erythrocyte porphyrin results exclude the acute porphyrias principally variegate porphyria and hereditary coproporphyria and also the hepatic porphyria; porphyria cutanea tarda (PCT).

2. In PCT, the urinary PBG is not increased (remember that this is not one of the acute porphyrias), while the urinary total porphyrins are increased usually of the uro- and heptapor-phyrin types. The faecal total porphyrins are also increased, showing elevations of isocoproporphyrin and heptapor-phyrin. The plasma fluorescence peak is at 615 nm and of course the erythrocyte porphyrins would not be expected to be elevated. Porphyria cutanea tarda is thought to be the result of a defect in the enzyme uroporphyrinogen decar-boxylase. There are at least three varieties: the familial type which is inherited as an autosomal dominant; a sporadic type; and a toxic variant, often the result of halogenated hydrocarbon toxins. Liver function tests can frequently be abnormal.

3. Protoporphyria is an autosomal defect of ferrochelatase affect-ing about 1 in 200 000 individuals. Typically, urine PBG and urine total porphyrins are not increased and faecal porphyrins may only show a moderate elevation of protoporphyrin. The plasma and erythrocyte fluorescence emission peak shows a peak at 632 nm. Erythrocyte porphyrin determination shows a predominant increase in free protoporphyrin.

4. Lead poisoning can interfere with a number of steps in haem biosynthetic pathways. Although urinary PBG excretion can be increased, this occurs to a much lesser degree than 5-aminolaevulinate (ALA) which can be found in high concen-trations. Increased urine porphyrins, particularly in the form of coproporphyrin III, are also features of lead poisoning. Elevated erythrocyte total porphyrins are an additional biochemical finding, but unlike protoporphyria the zinc-protoporphyrin is the predominant type rather than free protoporphyrin. It is also worth mentioning that iron deficiency and sideroblastic anaemia can also result in increased erythrocyte porphyrins but usually of the free protoporphyrin variety.

Case 25

A 38-year-old policeman was referred to the endocrinologists because of suspected acromegaly by his GP. He complained of impaired peripheral vision which he had noticed when driving his patrol car down narrow streets. His wife had also noticed that his appearance had altered and that he had put on weight. Physical examination showed large hands and feet and his visual fields confirmed a peripheral field loss. Ophthalmoscopy showed optic atrophy. His blood pressure was 164/98 and a trace of glucose was found in his urine.

The GP had also sent off some preliminary biochemical tests, the results of which were sent to the endocrine clinic with the referral letter. Some of these results were as follows: calcium 2.58 mmol/l; phosphate 2.51 mmol/l: albumin 40 g/l; random venous plasma glucose 13.7 mmol/l.

Questions

1. What biochemical investigations could you perform to confirm the doctor's clinical suspicion of acromegaly?
2. One of the attending medical students in the endocrinology out-patients commented upon the phosphate result. What is the most likely explanation?
3. What are causes of hyperphosphataemia?

Answers

1. A useful dynamic test is the oral glucose tolerance test when in normal individuals the serum growth hormone (GH) concentration should reach undetectable amounts, usually less than 1 mU/l. In acromegalics, this suppression is not seen, and there may even be a paradoxical increase in serum GH. Perhaps less preferable, is the measurement of serum GH on four separate occasions spaced evenly throughout the day. Acromegalics maintain measurable GH in each sample, whereas normal subjects only show GH in half the samples. Random serum GH determinations are of little use because of the episodic secretion of the hormone. Recently, it has been suggested that elevated serum insulin-like growth factor 1

(IGF-1) occurs in acromegaly and that this could become the basis of a useful screening test.

Once the diagnosis has been confirmed, it is important to exclude impairment of pituitary function. An insulin tolerance test is usually necessary to measure the release of corticotrophin (ACTH), gonadotrophins (LH and FSH) and thyrotrophin (TSH). Remember that, in patients with elevated GH, the patient may need a larger insulin dose than is usual because of their relative insulin resistance, although all insulin stress tests should be performed with great care to avoid dangerous hypoglycaemia. These is also an association between acromegaly and the syndrome of multiple endocrine neoplasia (MEN) especially the MEN type 1 variety associated with parathyroid adenomas, pancreatic adenomas and adrenocortical adenomas.

2. Hyperphosphataemia is observed in some acromegalics. Excess GH secretion can result in decreased excretion of phosphate. Non-specific findings in acromegaly include increased urinary calcium excretion and impaired glucose tolerance or diabetes mellitus. The latter is evident in our patient. However, none of these observations are pathogonomic for acromegaly.

3. A common cause of artefactual hyperphosphataemia is haemolysis or an old blood specimen which has not been promptly handled to separate the plasma from the erythrocytes. Increased release of phosphate, which is predominately an intracellular anion, occurs in starvation, malignant hyperpyrexia, diabetic ketosis and acidosis. Sometimes, there is increased dietary intake of phosphate as may occur in infants fed unmodified cows' milk which can be high in phosphate. Vitamin D intoxication can also result in hyperphosphataemia. A common

Table 14 Some causes of hyperphosphataemia

Increased tissue breakdown, e.g. tumour lysis syndrome and malignant hyperpyrexia
Artefact due to haemolysis or old sample
Acute or chronic renal failure
Acidaemia
Diabetic ketoacidosis
Hypoparathyroidism
Acromegaly
Excess vitamin D
Inapproprately high phosphate intake, usually intravenously

cause of hyperphosphataemia in hospital patients is acute or chronic renal failure. Hyperphosphataemia may also occur with bony metastases, when phosphate is released from the bone, and as a result of hypoparathyroidism. *Table 14* lists some causes of hyperphosphataemia.

Case 26

A 10-year-old schoolboy was referred to the paediatric endocrine clinic because of short stature. He had undergone a normal birth and went on to achieve normal milestones. His health was unexceptional and he was taking no medication. He had no gastrointestinal symptoms and there was no family history of note. He seemed to be doing well at school apart from disliking attending because of bullying due to his size. His two brothers were also well; the eldest was 12 years with a height of 1.52 m and the youngest was 9 years with a height of 1.40 m. His father was 1.79 m tall and his mother 1.69 m. On physical examination, the boy's height was 1.16 m, yet his genitals were considered normal for his age. He had normal body proportions and his appearance was not abnormal. Examination of his nervous system was unremarkable and he had a normal sense of smell and no optic atrophy. No other abnormality could be detected including that of the thyroid gland. His weight was 40 kg and blood pressure 98/72.

Questions

1. Give some possible causes for this child's short stature.
2. How could this child be investigated?
3. Insulin-like growth factor 1 (IGF-1) has been used to assess growth disorders, but what factors can lower serum IGF-1 levels?

Answers

1. There are many causes of short stature in children. One should consider the following broad categories. Low birthweights,

familial tendency, chromosomal defects, constitutional delay, growth defects such as the dysmorphic or disproportion syndromes, nutritional problems, psychosocial problems, chronic ill health, musculoskeletal defects, and endocrine abnormalities.

2. The investigation of short stature depends somewhat upon the medical history and physical examination. Routine blood tests, including full blood count, liver, renal and thyroid function tests can be useful in screening for an underlying disease. Malabsorption states, including cystic fibrosis and coeliac disease, can manifest as disorders of stature. Chromosome analysis can also be of value if a chromosomal abnormality is suspected. Height measurements of other family members may also indicate familial growth disorders. It is also important to accurately record the patient's weight and height and to measure growth velocity and record results ideally on two separate occasions over a six-month to one-year period. Tanner-Whitehouse growth-charts are useful, particularly as a normal growth velocity despite short stature can be a feature of familial or constitutional growth problems. A nutritional assessment and a psychosocial history can also be useful, as can measuring the patient's bone age.

If multiple endocrine defects are found, including impaired gonadal development, pituitary function should be assessed, including pituitary scanning and a combined pituitary function test.

A number of tests are presently available to assess growth hormone status. Random serum growth hormone (GH) levels are not of much value because of the episodic nature of GH secretion and because the anterior pituitary gland's GH reserve is not being examined. A simple screening test is to take serial blood samples in the hope of detecting a serum GH of greater than 20 mU/l, which implies a normal pituitary GH response; but of course one may be unlucky and miss the correct sampling times. Stimulation tests for GH have therefore been advocated. These include oral amino-acids, in the form of Bovril, or exercise using a bicycle ergometer. These tests have been used as screening tests for GH deficiency but more definitive stimulation tests include intravenous or intramuscular glucagon, particularly in children under five years old or when the insulin tolerance test is contraindicated. Other stimulation tests include oral or intravenous clonidine or intravenous arginine. Sleep can also result in GH release and this physiological stimulus has been utilized as a stimulation test. The insulin tolerance test can be used to assess not only GH pituitary reserve, but also other pituitary hormones in situations where hypopituitarism is considered, although isolated GH deficiency is well described. A word of warning is necessary as this test should be closely monitored, bearing in mind contraindications to the test such as epilepsy and severe panhypopituitarism. Remember also that in cases of growth hormone deficiency, a lower dose of insulin may be needed than expected to induce hypoglycaemia. In peri-pubertal children, stimulatory tests can be equivocal and sex hormone priming can be performed before testing.

3. Basal serum insulin-like growth hormone 1 (IGF-1) concentration has been suggested as a good screening test for growth hormone defects. This compound regulates the response of GH at the tissue level by stimulating tyrosine kinase activity at its own IGF-1 receptor. Low serum levels imply GH deficiency and high serum concentrations are observed in acromegaly. Serum IGF-1 is a cost-effective screening test for GH deficiency, although low serum concentrations may occur in malnutrition states, thyroid deficiency, Cushing's syndrome, renal and liver disease, insulin deficiency and hypothermia. Interestingly, pygmies have abnormal IGF-1 synthesis and Laron dwarfs have a defect of the GH receptor and low IGF-1 levels.

Case 27

A 66-year-old retired lorry-driver was a regular attender of the hospital renal department because of his chronic renal failure (CRF) for which he received haemodialysis. The cause of his CRF was polycystic kidneys. He lived alone, his wife having died two years previously. He smoked 10 cigarettes per day and drank one pint of lager at the weekend. Unfortunately, his renal function was slowly deteriorating and he was complaining of increasing tiredness and weakness. His blood pressure was also worsening and measured 168/102. As usual, blood was sent to the clinical chemistry department before and after his dialysis. The most recent predialysis results were as follows: sodium 132 mmol/l; potassium 6.5 mmol/l; chloride 96 mmol/l; bicarbonate 13 mmol/l; urea 63.6 mmol/l; creatinine 0.79 mmol/l; calcium 1.96 mmol/l; phosphate 2.50 mmol/l; albumin 38 g/l; magnesium 1.80 mmol/l.

Questions

1. Comment upon the abnormal biochemical findings and the underlying pathophysiology.
2. Why is the plasma calcium concentration low?
3. Explain the plasma magnesium level.
4. What other conditions can give a similar plasma magnesium concentration?

Answers

1. This patient is in end-stage CRF. The plasma creatinine concentration of greater than 0.50 mmol/l implies that the glomerular filtration rate (GFR) in this patient has fallen to below 20 ml/min. It is useful to remember that, as a rough guide, the plasma creatinine concentration is proportional to the reciprocal of the GFR. This assumes that the amount of creatinine filtered at the glomerulus equals the amount excreted in the urine. This is only an approximation as about 10% of urinary creatinine is secreted by the proximal tubule. In severe CRF, this secretion increases. Since about 45% of urea filtered at the glomerulus is reabsorbed, the patient is clearly uraemic. There is recent evidence that high urea concentrations can be toxic.

   According to the intact nephron hypothesis, the biochemical findings seen in CRF can be explained by the assumption that although there is a progressive decrease in nephron number the remaining nephrons are fully functional. Both hydrogen ions and potassium ions are regulated by the kidneys partly by tubular control. In end-stage CRF, one usually observes retention of these compounds and consequently a metabolic acidosis and hyperkalaemia. Our patient displays both phenomena. Tubular reabsorption of sodium is generally decreased in CRF and this may partly explain the patient's hyponatraemia. However, there is also a concentrating defect of urine in CRF, with urine osmolality approaching that of plasma. This is called isosthenuria.

2. The hypocalcaemia is partly the result of a reduction in the renal activity of the enzyme 1-alpha hydroxylase. This enzyme is responsible for producing the active vitamin D metabolite, 1,25 dihydroxycholecalciferol. As a result of this defect, there is reduced intestinal calcium absorption. Another contributing factor for the hypocalcaemia is precipitation of calcium and phosphate complexes, due to hyperphosphataemia. The latter is the result of the declining GFR; about 90% of the filtered phosphate at the glomerulus is reabsorbed.

Remember that hypocalcaemia can cause the release of parathyroid hormone (PTH) in an attempt to normalize plasma calcium. This is termed secondary hyperparathyroidism. This may sometimes lead to a parathyroid adenoma, resulting in autonomous PTH secretion and tertiary hyperparathyroidism.

3. Hypermagnesaemia is observed in late-stage CRF due to impaired urinary excretion. Normally about 5% of the filtered magnesium at the glomerulus is excreted. Most is reabsorbed (60%) at the ascending loop of Henlé. There is evidence that PTH increases magnesium reabsorption. Hypermagnesaemia is important to recognize as it can result in muscle paralysis, coma, and bradycardia.

4. Apart from acute or chronic renal failure, hypermagnesaemia (*Table 15*) can be observed following excessive intake, whether orally, intravenously, or parenterally. Elevated plasma magnesium is sometimes seen immediately after magnesium administration for cardiac arryhthmias or myocardial infarction. Otherwise hypermagnesaemia is rare.

Table 15 Some causes of hypermagnesaemia

Acute or chronic renal failure
Inappropriate oral or intravenous magnesium administration
Sometimes in liver disease
Occasionally as a result of hypoxia
Hypocalciuric hypercalcaemia

Case 28

A 21-year-old squatter was brought to casualty because of an alleged drug overdose. He stated that he had consumed 20–30 paracetamol tablets about five hours previously because he was feeling 'fed-up'. He admitted also to being an intravenous drug abuser for the last five years with heroin being his main preference. Further questioning revealed he smoked 10 cigarettes per day and he drank seven pints of beer per week. He was on no medication and from his past medical history had been otherwise well, although he did say he had been admitted to hospital for hepatitis ten months previously. Physical examination showed a blood pressure of 110/72. There was nothing else of note, except for venepuncture scars on his arms, particularly near some tatoos.

His hospital notes were obtained from medical records, and these confirmed that he had been admitted ten months previously because of hepatitis B attributed to his intravenous drug habit. Induced emesis was performed and blood was taken for paracetamol and also liver function tests. The following results were obtained: paracetamol 20 mg/l; bilirubin 48 μmol/l; aspartate transaminase 221 U/l; alanine transaminase 376 U/l; alkaline phosphatase 434 U/l; albumin 34 g/l; total protein 101 g/l.

Questions

1. Comment upon his liver function tests.
2. Comment also about the paracetamol blood concentration in relation to hepatic damage.
3. What can be the biochemical features of a paracetamol overdose?

Answers

1. The liver function tests would be compatible with chronic hepatitis and with the knowledge that the patient had hepatitis B 10 months previously. Hepatitis lasting longer than six months is usually defined as chronic. Chronic hepatitis can be subclassified into chronic persistent (CPH) and chronic active (CAH) forms. This patient probably has the latter variety, in which there is often a moderate elevation of bilirubin and also of alkaline phosphatase indicating a degree of cholestasis; elevated plasma globulins (total plasma protein concentration – plasma albumin concentration) depicting a chronic inflammatory process; and moderate to severe elevation of transam-

inases due to hepatocyte necrosis. Note that his plasma albumin concentration is reduced implying a defect of hepatic synthesis, with the risk of progressing to cirrhosis. Although the diagnosis of CAH or CPH is usually differentiated by the histological findings at biopsy, CPH tends to manifest as elevated plasma transaminases but normal plasma albumin and globulin concentrations.

2. Assuming the patient is correct about the time of intake, the plasma paracetamol concentration of 20 mg/l suggests that hepatic damage is unlikely. However, remember that it is important not to sample for paracetamol plasma levels within four hours post-ingestion as absorption of the drug may be incomplete. Should there be any doubt regarding timing, the blood paracetamol assay should be repeated a few hours later to establish the amount and direction of the change. Action lines based upon plasma paracetamol concentrations plotted against time from ingestion have been published and are important in assessing the risk of hepatic damage.

   Patients who have plasma paracetamol levels indicative of hepatic risk may benefit from N-acetylcysteine therapy which repletes glutathione stores.

   Sometimes, there is the diagnostic problem of a patient for whom it is difficult to assess the time of sampling accurately. In these cases, it has been suggested that calculation of the plasma paracetamol half-life from the results of two serial samples taken four hours apart is of value. A half-life of more than four hours suggests either hepatic damage or possible saturation of the paracetamol-metabolizing enzymes. Remember also that if the patient is taking other drugs which are known to be enzyme-inducers or are themselves hepato-toxic (this includes ethanol), the risk of liver damage may be present at even lower plasma paracetamol concentrations.

3. Paracetamol is metabolized by conjugation with glucuronide and sulphate within the liver. A small amount is however, converted by mixed function oxidases to reactive metabolites which are toxic to cells. Under normal circumstances these metabolites are detoxified by glutathione but at high para-cetamol concentrations this pathway becomes fully utilized and toxicity results.

   The prothrombin time should be measured approximately 12-hourly in patients at risk, as this is probably the best marker of hepatic necrosis. Plasma bilirubin and the transaminases can also increase, with aspartate transaminase usually increasing by more than alanine transaminase. These changes are often noticed about 24–72 hours post-paracetamol ingestion.

Fulminant hepatic failure is heralded by an increasingly prolonged prothrombin time and very elevated plasma transaminases. There may also be disseminated intravascular coagulation with elevated fibrinogen degradation products, such as fibrin fragment B3 and fibrinopeptide A. Acute renal failure can also develop as can more rarely acute pancreatitis.

Case 29

A 39-year-old publican was seen in the casualty department because of abdominal pain that had persisted for at least five hours. This was worse in the epigastric region and radiated through to his back. He also complained of nausea. He stated that he had experienced similar episodes of abdominal pain over the previous six years, but that this attack was the most severe yet. He was not on any medication but he admitted to smoking 40 cigarettes per day and to drinking on average half a bottle of whisky per day. On examination, he had a blood pressure of 98/68, pulse of 98/min, and was very distressed because of the pain. He was very tender over his abdomen, particularly over the epigastric region. Blood was taken for emergency laboratory tests, with the following results: sodium 148 mmol/l; potassium 3.5 mmol/l; urea 13.2 mmol/l; creatinine 0.12 mmol/l; calcium 1.78 mmol/l; phosphate 0.81 mmol/l; albumin 31 g/l; bilirubin 12 μmol/l; alanine transaminase 58 U/l; alkaline phosphatase 232 U/l; gamma-glutamyl-transferase 221 U/l; amylase 5400 U/l; random venous plasma glucose 10.1 mmol/l. A full blood count showed a haemoglobin of 14.2 g/dl; white cells $16 \times 10^9/l$ and platelets $152 \times 10^9/l$.

Questions

1. What is this acute abdomen likely to be due to, and would this attack be considered severe?

2. What are other causes of an elevated serum amylase?

3. This man survived this abdominal emergency, but three years later he was referred to a gastroenterologist with weight loss, glycosuria, abdominal pain and steatorrhoea. What could be the diagnosis and what other biochemical investigations might confirm this?

Answers

1. The diagnosis was acute pancreatitis secondary to high ethanol consumption. About 10% of cases of acute pancreatitis are alcohol-related, although gall-stones are a common cause. Other causative agents are hyperlipidaemia, hypercalcaemia, trauma and certain drugs.

   This would be deemed a severe attack. In this patient, bad prognostic features based upon laboratory tests are hypocalcaemia below 2.0 mmol/l, a plasma albumin of less than 32 g/l, a glucose of greater than 10 mmol/l, and a white cell count of more than 15×10^9/l. Also prognostically bad are hypoxia, a plasma urea of greater than 16 mmol/l and elevated alanine transaminase of greater than 200 U/l. However, these prognostic scores are usually based upon the findings up to 48 hours after an attack. There remains a need for earlier biochemical prognostic markers for acute pancreatitis and some authors have suggested serum C-reactive protein (CRP), urinary albumin or urine trypsinogen activation peptides – all of which are elevated in an attack. The extent of the hyperamylasaemia, however, is not an indicator of the severity of pancreatic damage, as only moderate elevations can be seen in haemorrhagic pancreatitis or if there is little pancreatic tissue remaining.

2. Serum amylase is derived from two main sites, either the pancreas or the salivary glands. Unfortunately, other acute abdominal situations can cause an elevation of serum amylase, such as intestinal obstruction, mesenteric infarction, perforated duodenal ulcers and peritonitis (*Table 16*). Fallopian tube disorders can similarly result in hyperamylasaemia, as can certain tumours, notably lung and ovary. Drugs, including steroids and opiates, may raise serum amylase as can diabetic ketoacidosis. Amylase is a relatively small protein and as such is filtered into the urine.

   Elevations in serum amylase levels can occur in renal disease. This is an important principle as there is a variant

Table 16 Some causes of hyperamylasaemia

Acute pancreatitis
Intestinal pathology
• Intestinal obstruction
• Mesenteric infarction
• Perforated peptic ulcer
Ethanol or methanol intake
Renal disease
Salivary disease
• Mumps
• Calculi
Macroamylasaemia
Malignant disease

form of amylase called macroamylasaemia. In this condition, individuals show moderately elevated serum amylase but an absence of amylase in the urine because the amylase cannot be excreted in the urine. Macroamylasaemia can cause diagnostic confusion with acute pancreatitis. A urine amylase determination can help to distinguish between the two conditions, being low or undetected in the former, while in acute pancreatitis the urine amylase:creatinine ratio is high. Raised serum amylase can also result from salivary gland disease, e.g. mumps.

It can therefore be seen, that serum amylase is not very specific for acute pancreatitis, although very high levels over 2000 U/l are very suggestive of the condition. In view of this, other biochemical tests have been considered for facilitating the diagnosis of acute pancreatitis. Some possible alternatives include serum lipase determination, serum amylase isoenzymes, urinary amylase or amylase:creatinine ratios, or peritoneal fluid amylase.

3. In view of the patient's previous medical history, chronic pancreatitis should be considered. A faecal fat determination and the demonstration of hyperglycaemia are useful. Some have proposed measuring serum amylase or lipase after pancreozymin and/or secretin stimulation to assess pancreatic reserve. Others favour duodenal intubation studies, such as the Lundh test or pancreozymin and/or secretin stimulation in which the volume and concentrations of bicarbonate and pancreatic enzymes are measured in duodenal fluid. A tubeless test involving hydrolysis of oral synthetic tripeptide N-benzoyl-tyrosyl-aminobenzoic acid (NBT-PABA) by pancreatic

chymotrypsin has also been used. An indirect measurement of pancreatic function can be made by measuring released PABA excreted into the urine.

Case 30

A five-week male infant was referred to the teaching hospital paediatricians because of failure to thrive and vomiting which had been present for three weeks but without explanation. Apart from the first two days, the baby had been bottle-fed from birth and his growth was thought to be normal. He had one sister aged three years and there was no family history of note. Examination revealed hepatosplenomegaly. A number of blood tests were performed. Some of the results are presented here with age-related reference values in parentheses: bilirubin 62 μmol/l (<24); alanine transaminase 70 U/l (<45); albumin 32 g/l (30–45); prothrombin time 71 sec (11–16); alkaline phosphatase 2343 U/l (<1010); calcium 2.20 mmol/l (2.10–2.50); phosphate 1.0 mmol/l (1.40–2.25); haemoglobin 10.3 g/dl (9.5–12.5); white cells 12.3 × 10⁹/l (10–25); platelets 786 × 10⁹/l (150–450); serum alpha-fetoprotein (AFP) 180 000 KU/l (20–3400). Urine analysis revealed gross aminoaciduria.

Questions

1. What is the most likely diagnosis?
2. What other biochemical tests would you request to establish the diagnosis?

Answers

1. The diagnosis is tyrosinaemia type 1, also called tyrosinosis. This condition is an inborn error of metabolism inherited as an autosomal recessive, with an incidence of about 1 in 200 000, although there is an area of Canada where the incidence is as high as 1 in 2000. Typically, this condition presents in neonates

as diarrhoea, vomiting, failure to thrive, hepatomegaly and nephropathy with Fanconi syndrome. Also observed are increased prothrombin time and serum AFP, consistent with hepatic damage, and also thrombocythaemia or conversely thrombocytopenia.

Untreated this condition can lead to death in the first year of life usually from hepatic failure. A more chronic variety is observed in which 40% of cases develop hepatoma in the first two decades of life. Treatment has consisted of a low phenyl-alanine and tyrosine diet and liver transplantation. The enzyme defect is probably a deficiency of fumarylacetoacetate hydro-lase, which results in a toxic build-up of the metabolites succinylacetone and fumarylacetoacetate. Recently, there has been excitement about nitro-trifluoromethyl-benzoyl-cyclo-hexanedione (NTBC) a compound that prevents the formation of these toxic metabolites. Accumulation of these metabolites helps to explain some of the clinical sequelae of this disorder, as the metabolites have been shown to be nephrotoxic. This would account for the Fanconi syndrome (this patient has aminoaciduria and hypophosphataemia) and the hepatic damage reflected by abnormal liver function tests, including the prothrombin time.

Some patients can develop rickets as a result of the hypophosphataemia due to the Fanconi's syndrome. Also observed in some patients is an increase in plasma 5-amino-laevulinate (ALA), a precursor of porphyrin synthesis. This can be explained by the fact that succinylacetone also inhibits the enzyme porphobilinogen synthase.

Tyrosinaemia type 1 should not be confused with Richner-Hanhart syndrome or tyrosinaemia type 2 in which there is mental retardation, hyperkeratosis and eye problems, includ-ing conjunctivitis and keratitis. Although, similarly, there is increased plasma tyrosine, there is also increased urinary excretion of phenolic acid derivatives of tyrosine. The defect is thought to be of the enzyme tyrosine aminotransferase. Another defect of the amino acid tyrosine seen in neonates, is transient tyrosinaemia of infancy which is related to prematu-rity and high protein diets. This is caused by immaturity of the enzyme hydroxy-phenylpyruvate dioxygenase.

2. Plasma tyrosine is elevated in this disorder, often to levels over 500 μmol/l. Urinary succinylacetone can be measured by gas chromatography-mass spectroscopy and is usually grossly elevated. The diagnosis is further confirmed by finding a low

activity of the enzyme fumarylacetoacetate hydrolase in cultured fibroblasts. Serum AFP and liver function tests can be used to monitor treatment and also to indicate the development of hepatoma.

Case 31

A 20-year-old unemployed woman was seen in casualty because she claimed she had taken an overdose of aspirin about five hours ago. When asked about the number of tablets taken, she thought this totalled 40. She refused to explain why she had taken the tablets and also refused to answer any further questions, although she did admit to her ears ringing. Soon after her admission to casualty, she complained of nausea and vomited twice. On examination, she appeared flushed, was sweating and was clearly hyperventilating. Her blood pressure was 100/60.

Blood was taken for biochemical analysis and the following results were obtained: sodium 138 mmol/l; potassium 3.7 mmol/l; bicarbonate 20 mmol/l; chloride 108 mmol/l; random venous plasma glucose 4.5 mmol/l. Plasma paracetamol was undetected, but the plasma salicylate concentration was 2.8 mmol/l (450 mg/l). Blood gases were later sent for analysis, with the following results being obtained: pH 7.55; $PaCO_2$ 25 mmHg, PaO_2 100mmHg.

Questions

1. What is the acid/base disturbance?
2. What other acid/base disturbances can be seen with salicylate overdose?
3. What are causes of a respiratory alkalosis that can be seen in hospital patients?

Answers

1. The blood gas results show a respiratory alkalosis. As a result of increased alveolar ventilation the $PaCO_2$ decreases result-

ing in an alkalaemia. An attempt at partial compensation is made, mainly by the kidneys which decrease tubular bicarbonate reabsorption and decrease the excretion of hydrogen ions. The net result of this is to decrease plasma bicarbonate concentration. The accompanying cation with the increased renal bicarbonate excretion is sodium. A reduction in the intravascular volume with a corresponding increase in reabsorption of sodium chloride by the proximal tubules can also result. Hence, sometimes in a respiratory alkalosis, an increased plasma chloride concentration is observed. Salicylate can stimulate the respiratory centre in the brain and thus lead to hyperventilation and subsequently a respiratory alkalosis.

2. In children, salicylate is more likely to produce a metabolic acidosis than in adults. A number of mechanisms have been suggested, such as the uncoupling of oxidative phosphorylation by salicylate. Furthermore, as a result of vomiting and sweating (salicylates also increase the body temperature in high dosage), patients can become fluid-depleted, leading to dehydration and even acute renal failure. Severe poisoning can lead to hypovolaemic shock and intravascular haemolysis. The vomiting, sometimes associated with salicylate overdose, can lead to a hypokalaemic metabolic alkalosis as a consequence of loss of acidic gastric contents. Furthermore, there may be a hypersensitivity reaction to the salicylate, particularly with severe overdose which can lead to pulmonary oedema. In extreme cases, adult respiratory distress syndrome or 'shock lung' can result leading to a respiratory acidosis. Other metabolic sequelae include hyperglycaemia or hypoglycaemia and sometimes hepatic damage.

   Blood drug levels of salicylate are useful in patient management, although clinical signs of toxicity do not always mirror drug levels. Severe salicylate poisoning is usually considered to occur above a plasma concentration of 3.1 mmol/l (500 mg/l) when a forced alkaline diuresis may be indicated.

3. A respiratory alkalosis is caused by increased alveolar ventilation. This can result from pneumonia, asthmatic attack, pulmonary embolism, and artificial ventilation using mechanical ventilators (*Table 17*). Mechanisms resulting from an increased respiratory centre drive include septicaemia, anxiety states, pregnancy and hepatic failure. Other centrally mediated mechanisms include brain lesions, such as tumours, head injury or infections.

Table 17 Some causes of a respiratory alkalosis

Pulmonary causes	Asthma
	Pneumonia
	Congestive cardiac failure
	Sometimes with artificial ventilation
Respiratory centre causes	Anxiety states
	Drugs, e.g. salicylates, doxapram
	Cerebral disease, e.g tumours, infection
	Hepatic failure
	Septicaemia
	Pregnancy

Case 32

Thursday was the day the senior registrar in clinical chemistry authorized the laboratory results. In the space of a couple of hours he had found, quite by chance, three abnormal results to arouse his curiosity. These all involved the electrolytes and renal function tests. Intrigued he went back to the original blood samples and the request cards to seek an explanation. The following are the three results:

(1) The first was a blood sample that had 'routine pre-op hip replacement' written on the request form. The results were: sodium 136 mmol/l; potassium 8.4 mmol/l; urea 5.7 mmol/l; creatinine 0.11 mmol/l.

(2) The second was a blood sample that had 'post-op cholecystectomy' written on the request form. The results were: sodium 156 mmol/l; potassium 0.8: urea 1.2 mmol/l; creatinine 0.04 mmol/l.

(3) The third blood sample was from a patient with diabetes mellitus admitted unconscious via casualty. The results were: sodium 148 mmol/l; potassium 5.0 mmol/l; urea 9.8 mmol/l; creatinine 0.52 mmol/l.

Questions

1. Explain the abnormal results of the first blood sample.
2. Why are the results of the second patient abnormal?
3. Explain the abnormal renal function tests in the diabetic patient.

Answers

1. Such an elevated plasma potassium, particularly in a patient with apparently normal renal function tests, is highly suspicious. One should exclude a haemolyzed sample, an old sample, or a sample stored in a fridge. In the case of the latter, cold is known to reduce the activity of the sodium/potassium pump, leading to leakage of potassium out of the cells. This sample had been taken only one hour before analysis and had not been kept in the fridge. Furthermore, there was no haemolysis visible. In fact the senior registrar had guessed at what had happened and had phoned the house-officer about how the blood sample was taken. It transpired that the sample had been contaminated with potassium/EDTA, used as the anticoagulant for the haematology full blood count tubes. The house-officer had transferred blood from this tube to the lithium/heparin chemistry tube after venepuncture.
2. The presence of a low potassium concentration with low plasma urea and creatinine levels suggests contamination from a drip-arm intravenous infusion. In fact the elevated sodium concentration indicated that the offending intravenous fluid probably contains saline. On questioning the house-officer, it became apparent that a medical student had bled the patient, but the venepuncture site was from the same arm as a saline drip.
3 It is unusual to have a highly elevated plasma creatinine concentration yet only a moderately elevated plasma urea concentration. The senior registrar tested the plasma sample for ketones which were strongly positive. Ketones can interact with the colorimetric Jaffe creatinine assay to give a falsely elevated apparent concentration of creatinine. In fact, this patient was in diabetic ketoacidosis.

Case 33

A 72-year-old retired meat-porter was admitted under the care of the urologists for a transurethral resection (TURP) of his prostate gland. He had complained of hesitancy upon micturition with nocturia for the previous six months. He smoked 12 cigarettes per day, drank six pints of beer per week and was taking bendroflurazide for hypertension. According to his past medical history, he had had one previous operation for an inguinal hernia 10 years ago, while in his teens he had suffered from rheumatic fever. On physical examination, his blood pressure was 146/92, but otherwise there was nothing else of note, apart from the rectal examination which revealed an enlarged prostate gland. His preoperative biochemistry tests showed: a sodium of 143 mmol/l; potassium 3.7 mmol/l; urea 7.6 mmol/l; creatinine 0.13 mmol/l; random venous plasma glucose 6.1 mmol/l.

The operation was an apparent success but the house-surgeon was alarmed to find the following biochemistry results after the operation: sodium 117 mmol/l; potassium 4.0 mmol/l; urea 5.6 mmol/l; creatinine 0.09 mmol/l.

Questions

1. Explain possible reasons for the hyponatraemia.
2. What are the other causes of hyponatraemia in hospital patients?
3. The histology of the tissue excised at the TURP showed malignant changes within the prostate gland. What biochemical tests can help in the diagnosis and management of prostatic carcinoma?

Answers

1. Postoperative hyponatraemia can be multifactorial. For example, inappropriate fluid replacement can result in haemodilution and hyponatraemia. Furthermore, as a result of pain, nausea and drugs given at operation, the secretion of antidiuretic hormone (ADH) can be increased and this can result also in hyponatraemia. However, this man has quite severe hyponatraemia and so other or additional explanations should be considered. In fact during surgery, the bladder was irrigated with glycine solution to prevent blood clots from blocking the urinary tract. It is now well recognized that large amounts of this hypotonic fluid can enter the circulation by passing through the prostatic vasculature bed, resulting in a dilutional hyponatraemia.

2. Hyponatraemia is a common biochemical abnormality in patients and can have many aetiologies (*Table 18*). Pseudohyponatraemia should always be excluded, such as can occur in hyperlipidaemia or paraproteinaemia. Excess solute in the extracellular space, as might occur with hyperglycaemia or mannitol therapy, should also be considered, as movement of intracellular water out of cells into the plasma will lead to a dilutional hyponatraemia. A condition called the 'sick cell syndrome' has also been proposed, whereby a defect of the sodium/potassium pump results in sodium influx into cells.

A useful classification is to categorize the hyponatraemia according to the extracellular fluid volume which can be clinically assessed, i.e. hypovolaemic, euvolaemic or hypervolaemic. Hypovolaemic hyponatraemia is often caused by a reduction in total body sodium and water, as occurs with vomiting, diarrhoea, burns, sweating and fistulae. In these cases, a urinary sodium concentration is usually less than 10 mmol/l. Other causes would include those involving renal loss of sodium and water, such as the use of diuretics, salt-losing nephropathies and mineralocorticoid deficiency (Addison's disease).

The euvolaemic hyponatraemia group can consist of hypothyroidism and chronic renal failure, and includes the syndrome of inappropriate antidiuretic hormone (SIADH). This condition can be due to the ectopic secretion of ADH by tumours (classically lung oat-cell carcinomas), chest disease such as pneumonia, asthma or intermittent positive pressure ventilation or head injury, meningitis or cerebrovascular accidents. Drugs should

Table 18 Some causes of hyponatraemia

Pseudohyponatraemia	Hyperlipidaemia/hyperproteinaemia
dilutional	Bladder irrigation with hypotonic fluid
	Hyperglycaemia
	Mannitol
Euvolaemic group	Syndrome of inappropriate ADH or inappropriate diuresis, e.g. malignancy, cerebral disease, pulmonary disorders, certain drugs, Hypothyroidism
Sodium loss group	Excess sweating, diarrhoea, vomiting
(usually hypovolaemic)	renal loss of sodium, e.g. diuretics, renal tubular acidosis, osmotic diuresis, mineralocorticoid deficiency
Hypervolaemic group	Sometimes in acute or chronic renal failure
	Hepatic cirrhosis, congestive cardiac failure, nephrotic failure (secondary hyperaldosteronism)

also be considered in this group and include vincristine, carbamazepine, narcotics, chlorpropamide and chlorpromazine. Some workers have suggested that a diagnosis of SIADH requires a number of criteria to be fulfilled, namely:

- Decreased plasma osmolality.
- High urine osmolality relative to plasma.
- Euvolaemia.
- High urinary sodium concentration (often taken as greater than 20 mmol/l).
- Absence of adrenal, renal, thyroid and hepatic malfunction.
- Increasing plasma sodium concentration upon water restriction.
- An elevated plasma ADH. In practice, ADH plasma assay is rarely performed.

It has also been proposed that there is a condition of cerebral salt wasting or a 'resetting of the body's osmostat'.

The hypervolaemic hyponatraemia group include oedematous states associated with secondary hyperaldosteronism. This hyponatraemic group consists of congestive cardiac failure, nephrotic syndrome and cirrhosis.

3. Serum prostatic acid phosphatase (PAP) and serum prostate specific antigen (PSA) can be used in aiding either the diagnosis of prostatic carcinoma or monitoring the response to therapy. Serum PAP and PSA can both be elevated in patients with benign prostatic hypertrophy (BPH). However, in the diagnosis of prostatic carcinoma, serum PSA is more sensitive but less specfic than serum PAP. Prostate carcinoma has a tendency to spread to bone and this is often heralded by an elevation in serum alkaline phosphatase (bone isoenzyme). It has also been stated that serum PSA is particularly elevated in the event of carcinoma spread to the retroperitoneal lymph nodes.

Case 34

A four-month-old female infant had been referred from a district general hospital to the university teaching hospital for investigation of feeding difficulties, hypotonia, convulsions and lethargy. She had been bottle-fed since birth as her mother had not believed in breast-feeding. She was the only child and her mother, who was adopted, was not aware of any familial disorders. Physical examination of the infant showed hypotonia and confirmed a somewhat lethargic baby. Some preliminary laboratory investigations showed: plasma sodium 136 mmol/l; potassium 3.5 mmol/l; bicarbonate 10 mmol/l; chloride 91 mmol/l; urea 5.5 mmol/l; creatinine 0.06 mmol/l; ammonia 447 μmol/l, random venous plasma glucose 3.5 mmol/l. Plasma amino acid determination showed increased concentrations of glycine. Urine analysis showed the presence of ketones, and specialized analysis by the paediatric laboratory found methylmalonic acid in the urine.

Questions

1. What is the metabolic disorder and what group of inherited diseases does this belong to?
2. What other causes of an elevated plasma glycine can be seen in clinical practice?

Answers

1. The urinary methylmalonic acid elevation should give this condition away as being methylmalonic acidaemia, one of the organic acidurias. This latter term has been used to define an increased urinary excretion of the acidic metabolites of fats, carbohydrates and amino acids. Many different organic acidurias have now been described largely due to the introduction of gas-liquid chromatography combined with mass-spectroscopy to detect organic acid metabolites. The child presented here has methylmalonic acidaemia, probably the commonest of these disorders. The condition is heterogeneous in that more than one enzyme defect has been described. One form is thought to be due to a deficiency of D-methylmalonyl-CoA racemase, another a defect of L-methylmalonyl-CoA mutase. Indeed, at least four other variants have been described. The situation is further complicated by the fact that methylmalonic acidaemia can also result from vitamin B_{12} deficiency and has even been reported in the breast-fed babies of strictly vegetarian mothers.

This child presents with many of the classic findings of methylmalonic acidaemia, namely hyperammonaemia, ketouria and a metabolic acidosis. Interestingly, thrombocytopenia and neutropenia have also been described. Mental retardation is a feature as is renal failure which is worsened by the accumulation of uric acid. Renal tubular potassium loss has also been described, leading to hypokalaemia.

There are many different organic acidurias and they will not all be listed here. However, some of the well-characterized ones are branched-chain ketoaciduria, isovaleric acidaemia and proprionic acidaemia. Some advances in prenatal diagnosis have been made, including metabolic analysis of amniotic fluid and also of maternal urine.

2. Hyperglycinaemia is a common finding in the organic acidaemias. This has also been observed in patients taking the antiepileptic drug, sodium valproate. Total parenteral nutrition is another cause. Other conditions worth bearing in mind are iminoglycinuria, prolinaemia and hydroxyprolinaemia. These metabolic disorders have increased plasma levels of hydroxyproline and/or proline. Finally, non-ketotic hyperglycinaemia is a condition in which the plasma/CSF ratio of glycine is increased.

Case 35

A 43-year-old baker was referred to the hospital lipid clinic because his GP had found abnormal blood lipid results during a well-man's screening clinic. The referring letter mentioned a fasting blood cholesterol of 9.8 mmol/l and triglycerides of 8.7 mmol/l. The patient described himself as essentially a well man, but admitted to pain in the calves when he walked more than 200 yards on the flat. He smoked 10 cigarettes per day and consumed about six units of alcohol per week. In his past medical history, he had no serious illnesses and no operations apart from a vasectomy three years previously. He had three children under 10 years of age who were well. Both his parents had died in their 60s but he was not sure for what reason. He had no brothers or sisters.

On examination, he was overweight with a body mass index of 27.1 and blood pressure of 146/90. The other significant findings were the absence of palpable foot pulses in both legs and there were yellow palmar striae on each of his hands. Resting ECG was normal, but Doppler ultrasound of his legs confirmed peripheral vascular disease.

Questions

1. What is the lipid abnormality?
2. Discuss biochemical investigations that may clarify the diagnosis.

Answers

1. This patient almost certainly has type III hyperlipidaemia, also known as broad beta-hyperlipidaemia because of the characteristic serum lipoprotein electrophoretic pattern often observed. The underlying biochemical defect is reduced clearance of chylomicron and very-low-density lipoprotein (VLDL) remnants. The palmar striae are considered pathognomic for the disorder, but tuberoeruptive xanthomata typically on the elbows and knees, xanthelasma and corneal arcus have also been described in this condition. Peripheral vascular disease is a typical feature of this hyperlipidaemic disorder, as is premature coronary artery disease. Classically, both serum cholesterol and triglyceride levels are about 9–10 mmol/l.

   Type III hyperlipidaemia should not be confused with familial combined hyperlipidaemia, a hyperlipidaemic condition in which there can be elevations of both serum cholesterol and triglyceride and which is also associated with premature cardiovascular disease. In this condition, variable lipid phenotypes can be expressed, either with a predominance of serum cholesterol (type IIa Frederickson's), hypertriglyceridaemia (type IV or V Frederickson's) or a combination of the two, i.e a mixed picture (e.g. type IIb Frederickson's). It has been postulated that this disorder is the result of increased synthesis of the apolipoprotein B100.

2. Serum lipid determination will frequently reveal hypercholesterolaemia and hypertriglyceridaemia, often in similar molar

proportions with serum concentrations of around 9 mmol/l. Serum levels of high-density lipoprotein (HDL) cholesterol are usually low.

Serum lipoprotein electrophoresis can show the classic type III picture with a broad beta-band composed of remnant particles. A homozygous association of type III broad beta-hyperlipidaemia with apolipoprotein(apo) E2 has been described, and thus apoE-phenotyping by a specialized laboratory can be useful, although some patients with broad beta-hyperlipidaemia can show other apoE phenotypes. Another investigation that can be useful in establishing the diagnosis is ultracentrifugation to separate the lipoprotein particles. The cholesterol of the VLDL particles is then quantitated and expressed as a total of the serum triglyceride concentration. In molar terms normal individuals show a ratio below 0.30, while ratios approaching 0.60, are more likely in broad beta-hyperlipidaemia.

It is becoming apparent that important as inheriting the apoE2 phenotype might be in developing broad beta-hyperlipidaemia, there may also be a triggering factor such as diabetes mellitus, hypothyroidism or obesity. These can be reasonably easily excluded by the clinical findings and appropriate biochemical tests, such as blood glucose determination and thyroid function tests. One should also be aware that systemic lupus erythematosus and multiple myeloma can produce a hyperlipidaemia similar to broad beta-hyperlipidaemia.

Case 36

A 3-year-old boy was sent to the paediatric out-patient clinic because of abdominal distension and hepatomegaly. The clinical history revealed that the child had become progressively unwell over the last six months with abdominal pain and tiredness. The boy was an only child and there was no family history of relevance. Physical examination confirmed severe hepatomegaly, as well as evidence of growth retardation. There was no muscle weakness or cardiomegaly. A number of blood tests were sent as an initial diagnostic screen, as the consultant paediatrician had a diagnosis in mind. Some of the non-fasting biochemistry tests were as follows: sodium 142 mmol/l; potassium 3.8 mmol/l; bicarbonate 15 mmol/l; chloride 101 mmol/l; urea 4.5 mmol/l; creatinine 0.06 mmol/l; urate 0.63 mmol/l; random venous plasma glucose 2.0 mmol/l; lactic acid 6.5 mmol/l; cholesterol 5.9 mmol/l; triglyceride 7.9 mmol/l.

Questions

1. What was the diagnosis the paediatrician had in mind?
2. Suggest further investigations to confirm the diagnosis.
3. Give other causes of an elevated plasma lactic acid.

Answers

1. The biochemical results and the hepatomegaly suggested to the paediatrician that she was dealing with a glycogen storage disease. This child was later shown to have Von Gierke's disease or type 1 glycogen storage disease. Further explanation of the biochemical features displayed here is necessary. The hepatomegaly is consistent with accumulation of hepatic glycogen granules that cannot be utilized. This leads to a shortage of glucose, and thus the hypoglycaemia as glycogenolysis is impaired. Alternative substrates are mobilized for energy requirements, including fats, which explains the hypertriglyceridaemia often encountered. The metabolic defect in von Gierke's disease is a deficiency of the enzyme glucose-6-phosphatase, which leads to a build-up of its substrate glucose-6-phosphate. This excess is channelled down the metabolic pathways of uric acid synthesis, resulting in the hyperuricaemia often observed. The increased glycolytic activity results in a lactic acid excess. Note also the metabolic acidosis depicted by the biochemistry results, as evidenced by the low plasma bicarbonate concentration and increased anion gap.
2. Diagnostic confirmation can be made by a liver biopsy and assay of the deficient enzyme. However, sometimes a glucagon stimulation test is useful. This tests works on the principle that phosphorylase is activated by glucagon which initiates glycogen degradation and subsequent further accumulation of glucose-6-phosphate. If plasma lactic acid is measured at baseline fasting, then at 30 and 45 minutes' post-glucagon

administration, a slight increase in plasma glucose is seen as well as a moderate increase in plasma lactic acid.

As an aide-memoire, the other glycogen storage diseases are:

(1) Type II or Pompé's disease due to 1,4 glucosidase deficiency and which is associated with hypotonia and cardiomegaly.

(2) Type III or Cori's disease due to a deficiency of amylo-1,6 glucosidase, which can be similar in presentation to type 1, except that hypoglycaemia is unusual.

(3) Type IV or Anderson's disease is due to amylo-transglucosidase deficiency.

(4) Type V or muscle phosphorylase deficiency or (McArdle's disease) results in muscle pain and weakness worse on exercise.

(5) In addition, there are other variants of glycogen storage disease, such as Her's disease.

3. In normal subjects, plasma lactate is usually less than 1 mmol/l and is a product of anaerobic glycolysis. If the blood pH is less than 7.25 and the plasma lactate concentration exceeds 5 mmol/l, then lactic acidosis is present. This is a form of metabolic acidosis associated with a raised anion gap and a low plasma bicarbonate concentration. Hyperlactaemia can result from severe muscle exercise when plasma concentrations exceed 20 mmol/l. Cohen and Woods devised a classification for lactic acidosis (*Table 19*):

(a) Type A is the result of tissue hypoxia and includes shock and hypovolaemic states, respiratory failure and severe anaemias.

(b) Type B is lactic acidosis occurring in the absence of hypoxia. This has been subclassified into type B1 due to either muscle damage, liver disease, deficiency of vitamin B_1 or excessive tumour glycolytic activity. Type B2 is drug-induced or poison-induced lactic acidosis, such as due to salicylates, methanol, ethanol, phenformin and ethylene glycol. Type B3 includes enzyme deficiencies that can lead to lactic acidosis. Examples include glycogen storage diseases, mitochondrial defects, and deficiency of fructose 1,6-diphosphatase.

(c) For those small print experts, a rare form of lactic acidosis involving *D*-lactate (as opposed to the more usual *L*-lactate varieties described above) is sometimes observed after small intestine resection and subsequent bacterial overgrowth.

Table 19 Some causes of lactic acidosis

Type A	Tissue hypoxia, e.g hypovolaemic or cardiogenic shock
	Hypotension
	Cardiac arrest
Type B1	Hepatic/renal/pancreatic disease
	Infections
	Tumours
Type B2	Biguanides
	Ethanol/methanol
	Salicylates
	Sorbitol or fructose administration
Type B3	Pyruvate decarboxylase deficiency
	Glycogen storage disease type 1
	Cytochrome c oxidase deficiencies
D-lactic acidosis	Small intestine bacteria production

Case 37

A 46-year-old company director attended a company health screening clinic. He claimed to be 'on the top of the world' regarding his health and thought there were no serious diseases running in his family. He admitted to smoking 30 cigarettes per day and to drinking three glasses of wine per week. He was taking no medication. On examination he had a blood pressure of 144/94 and a body mass index of 27.2. Otherwise, there was nothing else of note except that the patient looked slightly jaundiced. Resting ECG and chest X-ray were normal and a few routine blood tests were sent to the laboratory. The results of some of these tests are as follows: alkaline phosphatase 184 U/l; alanine transaminase 32 U/l; gamma-glutamyl transferase 34 U/l; albumin 42 g/l; bilirubin 55 μmol/l.

Questions

1. What differential diagnosis would explain these results?
2. What further tests would help establish an explanation for these findings?

Answers

1. A slightly elevated bilirubin in an otherwise healthy individual
   with normal liver function tests raises the possibility of Gilbert's
   syndrome. This condition, which has a normal life-expectancy,
   is thought to be due to reduced glucuronyl transferase activity. Some reports put the prevalence as high as 5% of the
   population and it has been proposed that the 'syndrome' may
   just reflect the upper end of the population's plasma bilirubin
   distribution. The diagnosis is largely one of exclusion to differentiate it from serious liver disease.

   The jaundice is usually not severe, being less than 100
   µmol/l. It often worsens upon fasting, viral infection or menstruation. The condition is frequently asymptomatic and is usually
   detected by routine blood testing or when the patient seeks a
   doctor for other reasons.

   Hyperbilirubinaemia is usually either the result of increased
   red cell destruction, as in haemolysis, or due to a liver or
   biliary abnormality. Some author's discuss hyperbilirubinaemia in terms of jaundice based upon an anatomical classification: pre-hepatic jaundice due to non-hepatic causes,
   usually haemolysis; hepatic jaundice due to hepatocellular
   disorders, and post-hepatic jaundice due to cholestasis, i.e
   biliary obstruction.

   A further helpful classification is to determine whether the
   hyperbilirubinaemia is due to predominantly unconjugated or
   conjugated bilirubin (*Table 20*). The predominantly unconjugated group consists of the haemolytic anaemias, Gilbert's
   syndrome, physiological jaundice of the newborn, breast-milk
   jaundice, the Crigler-Najjar syndrome (type 1 and 2), and the
   result of shunt or intravascular haemolysis.

   The predominantly conjugated group includes inherited
   disorders, such as Rotor's syndrome and Dubin-Johnson
   syndrome. Generally speaking, hepatocellular or cholestatic
   disease also produces mainly a conjugated hyperbilirubinaemia, although sometimes a mixed hyperbilirubinaemia is
   seen, i.e unconjugated bilirubin is present in the plasma as
   well as the conjugated form. Hepatitis, hepatotoxins, cirrhosis
   and metabolic liver disorders are examples of the former type,
   while cholestatic disease can result from either intrahepatic or
   extrahepatic causes. Unlike jaundice due to haemolysis, the
   hyperbilirubinaemia associated with hepatocellular defects is
   associated with bilirubin in the urine. Conversely the jaundice

Table 20 Some causes of hyperbilirubinaemia

Predominantly unconjugated	Haemolysis
	Gilbert's syndrome
	Physiological jaundice of neonates
	Crigler-Najjar type 1 or 2
	Rifampicin
	Congestive cardiac failure
	Occasionally, breast-feeding
Predominantly conjugated	Cholestasis
	Hepatitis
	Cirrhosis
	Liver infiltrations
	Hepatic toxins
	Metabolic hepatic disease
	Hepatotoxic drugs
	Rotor's syndrome
	Dubin-Johnson syndrome

of almost complete biliary obstruction results in the near-absence of bilirubin in the gut with the consequent lack of urobilinogen in the urine. Cholestasis is associated with elevated serum alkaline phosphatase activity.

2. To confirm the diagnosis, some of the above causes of hyper-bilirubinaemia should be excluded by the medical history or physical examination. A careful drug history is important as many drugs can cause liver disease, and rifampicin and some contrast media can give rise to an unconjugated hyperbiliru-binaemia. Clearly, to establish the diagnosis of Gilbert's disease, it must first be established that the bilirubin is predominantly unconjugated (almost synonymous with indirect bilirubin). Other hepatic function tests should be normal, including liver enzymes, plasma albumin and clotting studies. Haemolysis should also be excluded by a full blood count and film, reticulocyte count and haptoglobins.

In making the diagnosis, it helps if the unconjugated hyper-bilirubinaemia has been present in a well patient for six months without a worsening of liver function tests. In practice, however, the diagnosis is not so easy and more serious pathol-ogy sometimes needs to be excluded. Some laboratories measure fasting serum bile acids which are normal in Gilbert's syndrome but often elevated in hepatic disease. Others choose dynamic tests, such as the prolonged three-day fast, which results in an elevated plasma bilirubin in Gilbert's syndrome, or use intravenous nicotinic acid stimulation. Only in very difficult unclear cases would liver biopsy be considered in view of its potential risks.

Case 38

A 40-year-old mechanic presented to his general practitioner complaining of joint pain and nausea. On further questioning, it transpired that the symptoms had been getting worse over the last six months, and that recently the patient had also become impotent. The patient was a smoker of 15 cigarettes per day and drank about five pints of beer per week. In the last two months, he had reduced his beer intake because of nausea. He was on no medication except for paracetamol for his joint pain. Physical examination revealed a blood pressure of 138/88 and body mass index of 24.6. The general practitioner thought he looked 'suntanned' and also noted that he had hepatomegaly. The practice nurse noted glucose in his urine. The general practitioner took blood samples for laboratory testing and the following results were obtained: albumin 34 g/l; alanine transaminase 248 U/l; aspartate transaminase 221 U/l; bilirubin 44 µmol/l; alkaline phosphatase 384 U/l; random venous plasma glucose 12.9 mmol/l.

Questions

1. What is the most likely diagnosis?
2. What biochemical investigations would help to confirm the diagnosis?
3. Why is serum alpha-fetoprotein (AFP) used in the management of these patients?

Answers

1. The diagnosis that the general practitioner suspected was idiopathic haemochromatosis. This is an inherited condition

and shows an association with HLA-antigens, particularly A3 and B14. Evidence suggests that increased iron absorption results in excess deposition of iron into various tissues.

The presentation of diabetes mellitus, arthritis and gonadal dysfunction are characteristic of the condition, as is hypopituitarism and adrenal and cardiac defects. The condition was once called 'bronzed diabetes' because of the melanin pigmentation seen in these patients.

This patient also shows biochemical features of cirrhosis. There is elevation of the serum transaminases reflecting hepatocyte necrosis as well as an elevated alkaline phosphatase suggestive of cholestasis. Furthermore, the low serum albumin points to some degree of hepatic decompensation as there is impaired protein synthesis.

2. In this condition, the diagnosis is facilitated by measuring the serum iron, total iron-binding capacity (TIBC) and ferritin. The serum iron concentration is usually elevated with a high iron saturation (often greater than 75%), and the serum ferritin is usually grossly elevated. These tests do not always distinguish between the other iron overload states which include transfusion haemosiderosis, alcoholic secondary haemochromatosis and haemosiderosis due to haemolytic or sideroblastic anaemias. A liver biopsy can be used to confirm the diagnosis when an increase in hepatic iron stores (stainable with Prussian blue) is observed. This patient's serum iron was shown to be 40 μmol/l, TIBC of 42 μmol/l, iron saturation 96% and ferritin 1680 μg/l. Remember also that other forms of cirrhosis can lead to a high iron saturation, but this is partly because there is a decrease in transferrin production and thus a reduction in TIBC. Similarly, in severe haemochromatosis with advanced cirrhosis, the TIBC may be low with a normal serum iron concentration. It is also important to remember that ferritin is a positive acute-phase protein and can be elevated in malignancy, infections and hepatic disorders.

Other biochemical tests that may be abnormal in cirrhosis include increased immunoglobulins. For example, IgA is increased in early cirrhosis. Increased gamma-glutamyltransferase and plasma bile acids may also occur. There are also defects of the clotting pathways as the vitamin K-dependent clotting factors II, VII, IX and X are synthesized in the liver. These may be reflected by an increase in the prothrombin time.

In haemochromatosis, other biochemical tests may be directed at assessing the damage to other tissues, such as pituitary, adrenal and gonadal function tests. Furthermore, family members should also be screened by using serum ferritin, iron, iron saturation and TIBC. Some have suggested that ferritin determination should be the method of choice for screening, while others have proposed that iron saturation changes early in the course of the disease. Treatment consists of venesection and the iron-chelating agent desferrioxamine. This treatment is usually monitored using serial serum ferritin measurements.

3. One of the most severe complications of cirrhosis is hepatoma. Serum AFP can be used as a tumour marker. Normal serum concentrations are below 10 KU/l, although these sometimes reach 500 KU/l due to hepatic regeneration, as can be seen in hepatitis and cirrhosis. However, most hepatomas result in a serum AFP concentration above 500 KU/l and occasionally above 10 000 KU/l.

Case 39

A 41-year-old teacher presented to her general practitioner complaining of weight loss and diarrhoea. She was not on any medication, was a non-smoker, drank only an occasional glass of wine, and had never had any serious illnesses. However, there was a family history of cardiovascular disease. Her father died of a myocardial infarction at the age of 42 years and a brother had started experiencing angina pectoris at the age of 49. On examination, she looked thin and manifested a tremor of her hands, her blood pressure was 128/76, and her radial pulse was 96/min. Her thyroid was diffusely enlarged with a bruit to auscultation. Examination of her eyes revealed slight lid retraction. Otherwise the rest of the general practitioner's examination was normal. Suspecting thyroid disease, he arranged for thyroid function tests. In view of the family history of heart disease, a lipid screen was also performed. The following results were phoned back to him by the clinical chemistry laboratory: TSH <0.05 mU/l; fT4 43 pmol/l; fT3 23 pmol/l; random cholesterol 2.0 mmol/l.

Questions

1. The diagnosis should be obvious. What is it?
2. Comment upon the serum cholesterol result.
3. What conditions can give a similar serum cholesterol result?
4. Discuss causes of a low HDL-cholesterol.

Answers

1. The classic signs upon examination and the suppressed TSH and elevated fT4 and fT3 point to a diagnosis of thyrotoxicosis or hyperthyroidism. This was caused by Grave's disease in this lady. The hyperthyroidism is thought to be due to the presence of thyroid-stimulating antibodies, whereas the ophthalmopathy is almost certainly due to ophthalmogenic immunoglobulins. The recent introduction of sensitive TSH assays has aided the diagnosis of hyperthyroidism because they allow suppression of serum TSH to be shown. The thyrotrophin-releasing hormone (TRH) test is less frequently used these days because of the improved TSH assays. In the TRH test, intravenous TRH fails to elicit a usual TSH response in hyperthyroid patients.

2. The serum cholesterol is low in this lady. This finding has been well described in hyperthyroidism but the explanation is not clear. However, thyroid hormones are important in cholesterol utilization by the tissues, as shown in hypothyroidism when an elevated serum cholesterol can be observed. Indeed, one of the older methods of lowering serum cholesterol was to use analogues of thyroxine, but this has now been replaced by safer medications.

3. Much is known about hypercholesterolaemic states but the converse is less clear. Severe liver damage, in the absence of cholestasis, can result in reduced serum cholesterol due to decreased synthesis. Starvation, end-stage uraemia, malabsorption states, malignant disease and certain anaemias can all result in a low or reduced serum total cholesterol concentration. Lipid-lowering drugs, including bile-salt binding resins, fibrates, nicotinic acid, and HMG-COA reductase inhibitors can all lower serum cholesterol, but so too can oestrogens, metronidazole and L-asparaginase. Hypocholesterolaemia has also been described in certain myeloproliferative diseases (*Table 21*).

Table 21 Some causes of hypocholesterolaemia

Total cholesterol	Starvation
	Tumours
	Myeloproliferative disease
	Severe hepatic disease
	Hyperthyroidism
	Severe sepsis
	Malabsorption states
	Sometimes in anaemias
	Cholesterol-lowering drugs
	Abetalipoproteinaemia (defect of apoB)
	Hypobetalipoproteinemia (defect of apoB)
HDL-cholesterol	Defects of apoA1 or A2
	Diabetes mellitus type II
	Insulin resistance (syndrome X)
	Chronic renal failure
	Obesity
	Androgens, some beta blockers, probucol
	LCAT deficiency
	Fish-eye disease

4. High-density lipoprotein (HDL) cholesterol has been of considerable recent interest because of the inverse relationship between HDL-cholesterol concentrations and coronary heart disease. Some clinicians now regard the total cholesterol:HDL-cholesterol ratio as more important than the total serum cholesterol in isolation in the assessment of cardiovascular risk factors. Low HDL-cholesterol states are generally defined as a serum concentration below 0.90 mmol/l. Also relevant is the fact that apolipoproteins (apo) A1 and A2 are important components of HDL particles and that HDL particles are heterogenous with HDL2 and HDL3 being predominant.

HDL-cholesterol is often decreased in hypertriglyceridaemic states, type II diabetes mellitus, obesity and chronic renal failure. Certain drugs, including probucol, some beta-blockers, androgens and corticosteroids, can lower HDL-cholesterol. Rare disorders causing a low HDL-cholesterol include familial lecithin:cholesterol acyltransferase (LCAT) deficiency, Tangier disease, fish-eye disease and disorders of apoA1 and A2.

Case 40

A 69-year-old lady visited her general practitioner because of tiredness and weakness. She complained that she had been getting progressively more tired over the last four months. On further questioning, it became apparent that she had also noted a change in bowel habit over the last six months. She was a non-smoker, drank little or no alcohol, and was taking a thiazide diuretic for hypertension. On examination, she looked clinically anaemic and her blood pressure was 148/88. Examination of her abdominal system was normal as was a digital rectal examination. The general practitioner took blood samples for a full blood count and thyroid function tests. In addition, she arranged for the patient to collect three faecal samples which she sent for occult blood analysis. A few days later, the results returned: TSH 1.6 mU/l; fT4 18 pmol/l; haemoglobin 9.2 g/dl; white cells 5.2×10^9/l, platelets 521×10^9/l, MCV 72 fl; MCHC 24g/dl. The occult bloods were all positive. In view of these findings, the general practitioner urgently referred the patient to the surgical outpatients, and in the interim sent further blood tests to the chemistry laboratory for serum iron, total iron-binding capacity (TIBC) and ferritin. The following results were obtained: iron 6 µmol/l; TIBC 72 µmol/l; ferritin 6 µg/l.

Questions

1. What type of anaemia is depicted?
2. Is this supported by the biochemistry results?
3. What is the significance of the positive faecal occult bloods?

Answers

1. The obvious anaemia with a microcytic, hypochromic blood picture and a low serum ferritin below 10 µg/l suggests an iron-deficiency anaemia. Such a pronounced hypochromia and micro-cythaemia are indicative of iron deficiency lasting at least a few months. A hypochromic anaemia is also seen in the anaemia of chronic disorders, i.e where there is a disturbance of the distribution of iron. In these cases ferritin tends to be elevated (or normal), due to it being a positive acute-phase protein.

2. The biochemical features presented here are typical of iron deficiency. The serum iron is low and the TIBC is high thus giving a low percentage iron saturation. The low serum ferritin suggests depleted iron stores. Remember that the TIBC is an indirect measure of transferrin, which is the major iron-carrying protein in plasma. Since one mole of transferrin binds two atoms of iron, then TIBC (μmol/l) divided by 2 is equal to the transferrin concentration (μmol/l). The transferrin saturation in healthy individuals is between 15–45%, but this declines to below 15% in iron deficiency. Whereas the TIBC is elevated in iron deficiency, it is reduced in the anaemia of chronic disease.

The problem with serum ferritin determination is that this protein is elevated by an acute phase response; thus results can sometimes be misleading when iron deficiency is suspected. This is in contrast to transferrin which is a negative acute phase protein. Serum iron alone is not a useful test as there is a considerable circadian variation in iron concentration. Some workers have proposed that erythrocyte protoporphyrin can be used diagnostically as this is increased in iron deficiency. This is due to impaired incorporation of iron into haem with consequent accumulation of protoporphyrin IX.

Some authors have classified iron deficiency into pre-latent, latent and frank iron deficiency. In the former, the body has a negative iron balance and there is enhanced iron absorption by the intestine. Clinical symptoms or signs of iron deficiency are usually absent. The blood haematology indices and serum iron and TIBC are within the reference range, although the serum ferritin can be reduced in some cases. In latent iron deficiency, the patient may complain of tiredness, although again the haematology results are usually within the reference range. However, serum iron is low and the TIBC elevated with a low serum ferritin. In frank iron deficiency, the patient is usually symptomatic with for example fatigue and may also show signs of chronic iron deficiency, such as glossitis and koilonychia. The haematology indices will be abnormal and the serum ferritin often below 15 μg/l.

3. It is not sufficient to simply make the diagnosis of iron deficiency without seeking an explanation for its presence. Some causes of iron deficiency are due to blood loss (50 ml of blood contains about 25 mg of iron), malabsorption states, increased iron requirements as in growth spurts, malignan-

cies, pregnancy, lactation and menstruation and reduced iron intake due to poor diet. The positive occult bloods in this patient suggest blood loss from the gastrointestinal tract as a cause of her iron deficiency. Indeed, it later transpired that the patient had a carcinoma of her caecum which was resulting in blood loss via the gut.

Case 41

A 17-year-old school-girl was seen in the medical out-patients because of weight loss. She had been well until the last year when she had lost about one stone in weight in a six month period. She had also stated that her periods were irregular and that over the last two months she had not menstruated. She had come off the oral contraceptive pill nine months ago because she had broken up from her boyfriend. In her past medical history, she had no operations and previously had been in good health. She was also a non-smoker and did not like alcohol. She was studying for her A-level exams and lived at home with her parents.

On examination she had a blood pressure of 100/60 and a body mass index of 23.1. She looked thin but had no signs of hyper-thyroidism. She had slight enlargement of her parotid glands and her dentition was poor. The rest of the examination was considered normal. A number of biochemical blood tests were sent and some of the following results were obtained: sodium 134 mmol/l; potassium 2.6 mmol/l; bicarbonate 45 mmol/l; chloride 82 mmol/l; urea 2.6 mmol/l; creatinine 0.09 mmol/l; random venous plasma glucose 3.4 mmol/l; TSH 2.1 mU/l; fT4 14.1 pmol/l. A pregnancy test was negative.

Questions

1. Comment upon the biochemical findings.
2. What would be a differential diagnosis?
3. What could be a possible explanation for the results in this patient?

Answers

1. The patient has hypokalaemia and also an elevated plasma bicarbonate with a low plasma chloride concentration. A high plasma bicarbonate can either be due to a metabolic alkalosis or a compensated respiratory acidosis. Subsequent blood gases in this patient showed a pH of 7.50, $PaCO_2$ of 47 mmHg and PaO_2 of 80 mmHg. These later results suggest an attempt by the body to compensate partially for the metabolic alkalosis by a reduction in pulmonary ventilation, thus resulting in an elevated $PaCO_2$.

2. The kidney has a remarkable capacity for excreting excess bicarbonate ions. To accumulate plasma bicarbonate, there must therefore be increased renal reabsorption of bicarbonate and/or an increase in bicarbonate production. The latter occurs in cases where hydrogen ions are lost from the body, as in vomiting of acid gastric contents or via the kidneys as seen in excess mineralocorticoid hormones (*Table 22*). Conversely, there can be an excessive intake of bicarbonate, as can occur with inappropriate administration of intravenous sodium bicarbonate or with the milk-alkali syndrome. Increased renal reabsorption of bicarbonate occurs in potassium depletion states, hypovolaemic states and mineralocorticoid excess, e.g. hyperaldosteronism, Cushing's syndrome and Bartter's syndrome.

3. The attending clinician noted the parotid and dental signs as well as the weight loss, all of which he considered consistent with pyschogenic vomiting, as in anorexia nervosa or bulimia. This would also explain the patient's metabolic alkalosis, hypokalaemia, and menstrual irregularity. However, he also considered Bartter's syndrome in his differential diagnosis. This defect is considered as one of the mineralocorticoid syndromes due to hyperplasia of the renal juxtaglomerular apparatus in which

Table 22 Some causes of a metabolic alkalosis

Increased bicarbonate intake	Inappropriate bicarbonate administration
	Milk-alkali syndrome
	High lactate or citrate intake
Hydrogen ion loss	Vomiting
	Chloride diarrhoea
Mineralocorticoid excess	
Severe hypokalaemia	

there is increased plasma renin activity and elevated plasma aldosterone. Low plasma potassium is noted along with a metabolic alkalosis in a patient who is often normotensive. However, on directly challenging the patient, she admitted to self-induced vomiting because she felt ugly and overweight, which was the reason, she thought, why her boyfriend had left her.

Urine chloride is a simple and useful way of classifying metabolic alkalosis. If the urine chloride concentration is less than 10 mmol/l, this suggests that the cause is either vomiting, chloride-losing diarrhoea, or excessive alkali intake. This group of causes for a metabolic alkalosis are termed saline-responsive, as a saline intravenous infusion can usually improve the alkalosis. However, if the urine chloride concentration is greater than 20–25 mmol/l, then this indicates either potassium deficiency or syndromes of mineralocorticoid excess, including Bartter's syndrome. In these cases, the term saline non-responsive metabolic alkalosis has been given and they are more likely to respond to potassium repletion. This patient had a urine chloride concentration of 6 mmol/l on a spot urine sample, thus further substantiating surreptitious vomiting.

Besides a hypokalaemic metabolic alkalosis, other biochemical features in patients with bulima or anorexia nervosa include elevations of liver enzymes, hypophosphataemia, hypomagnesaemia, and also hypercholesterolaemia. The liver enzyme abnormalities may be explained by fatty liver changes while the curious hypercholesterolaemia may be explained by decreased clearance of low-density lipoproteins. The hypokalaemia seen in patients with protracted vomiting is due to a combination of factors. Firstly, an alkalosis favours the uptake of potassium by cells. Secondly, small amounts of potassium are lost in the vomit. Finally, hypovolaemia, due to fluid loss, can lead to increased mineralocorticoid hormone secretion and thus increased potassium loss from the kidneys.

Case 42

A 45-year-old ex-secretary was under psychiatric care for manic-depression. She had been prescribed lithium about nine months previously and was initially seen regularly in the psychiatric day-hospital. Unfortunately, she started to avoid attending the hospital and she left the hospital catchment area without trace. Six months later, she reappeared at the same hospital complaining of feeling 'strange'. When asked she stated that she had taken her last lithium tablet about 12 hours previously. On examination, she had a blood pressure of 100/72, a pulse of 52 beats/min, and she looked overweight and lethargic. Blood was sent for thyroid function tests, electrolytes, renal function tests and serum lithium levels. The following results were obtained: sodium 145 mmol/l; potassium 4.3 mmol/l; urea 6.8 mmol/l; creatinine 0.11 mmol/l; TSH 14.6 mU/l; fT4 4.4 pmol/l; lithium 2.7 mmol/l.

Questions

1. Explain the thyroid function test results.
2. Comment upon the serum lithium concentration.
3. What are the features of lithium toxicity?

Answers

1. The elevated TSH and low free thyroxine (fT4) concentration indicate primary hypothyroidism. Lithium inhibits the release of thyroid hormones and can act as a goitrogen. Thyroid function tests should thus be regularly performed in patients on lithium therapy.
2. A serum lithium concentration of between 2.5–3.5 mmol/l, assuming that the patient was correct in her account of when she last took the drug, would indicate a considerable risk of severe intoxication. Oral lithium is rapidly absorbed with peak serum concentrations approximating to one hour post-dose. The half-life is between 8–20 hours. Steady state blood levels occur at about 3–7 days. As lithium has a long half-life, it is not usually necessary to measure serum levels within one week of altering the drug dosage unless of course toxicity is considered. Lithium has a narrow therapeutic window and inter-individual dosage requirements are surprisingly variable. In view of this, it has been recommended that blood samples for lithium determination are taken in the morning 12 hours after the evening dose, i.e. a trough level. The usual therapeutic range, based upon drug sampling at 12 hours' post-dose, is

between 0.30–1.30 mmol/l.

Potentially fatal intoxication should be considered with serum lithium levels greater than 3.5 mmol/l, while moderate poisoning is likely with serum concentrations between 1.5–2.5 mmol/l.

3. Apart from hypothyroidism, lithium toxicity can give rise to renal damage as well as nephrogenic diabetes insipidus. Thus patients may complain of polyuria and polydipsia. Lithium is 90% excreted by the kidneys and can undergo renal tubular secretion, with about 5% being eliminated in the sweat. Serum protein binding is minimal. Other features include nausea, vomiting and a leucocytosis. Effects upon the nervous system can also occur, such as seizures, ataxia, tremors, lethargy, nystagmus and dysarthria.

Plasma urea and creatinine determinations should also be monitored in patients on lithium as a pointer to early renal changes. Precipitating causes of lithium toxicity include impaired renal function, excessive acute lithium overdosage, or taking of lithium prescribed at too high a level. It was never clear with this patient how much lithium she had taken before her admission. Thiazide diuretics decrease renal secretion of lithium as does dehydration; conversely salt-loading increases lithium renal excretion. In severe cases, dialysis may be needed to control blood lithium levels.

Case 43

A 45-year-old schoolteacher was reviewed in the rheumatology clinic for her recently diagnosed Sjögren's syndrome. This had presented as joint aches in her limbs and swelling of her parotid glands. The best means of treating the syndrome was to be decided at this clinic visit. However, she complained of muscle weakness and lethargy. She had no diarrhoea and menstruation was normal for her. She was not taking any medication and was a non-smoker and only drank occasional alcohol at Christmas. There was nothing of note in her family history nor in her past medical history, except for a hysterectomy five years previously. In view of her weakness some blood tests were done and the results were as follows: sodium 143 mmol/l; potassium 2.8 mmol/l; bicarbonate 14 mmol/l; chloride 118 mmol/l; urea 6.8 mmol/l; creatinine 0.10 mmol/l; random venous plasma glucose 6.4 mmol/l.

Questions

1. What are the biochemical defects present?
2. Suggest a likely diagnosis.
3. What investigations can be useful in confirming this?

Answers

1. This patient has hypokalaemia and also a hyperchloraemic acidosis. A hyperchloraemic acidosis, also known as a normal anion gap acidosis, can be due to gastrointestinal loss of bicarbonate as in severe diarrhoea, ureteric diversion procedures and pancreatic fistulae (Table 23). Other causes include parenteral nutrition, hydrochloric acid ingestion, renal tubular acidosis, and use of the carbonic anhydrase inhibitor acetazolamide. Note that the plasma anion gap can be calculated by the following equation: (sodium + potassium) plasma concentrations – (chloride + bicarbonate) plasma concentrations.

   Normally this value is between 10–16 mmol/l, as is the case in this patient, although clearly her plasma bicarbonate concentration is low and the plasma chloride concentration is high.
2. From the patient's history a renal tubular acidosis (RTA) should be considered, particularly as the patient has Sjögren's

Table 23 Some causes of a hyperchloraemic acidosis

Renal tubular acidosis
Diarrhoea
Sometimes in renal failure
Sometimes in diabetic ketoacidosis after treatment
Ingestion of hydrochloric acid or ammonium chloride
Ureteric diversion such as ureterosigmoidostomy·
Drugs, such as carbonic anhydrase inhibitors or cholestyramine
Mineralocorticoid deficiency

syndrome which is associated with this condition. RTA is defined as a group of disorders in which there is a hyperchloraemic acidosis due to an abnormality of renal acid-base homeostasis. Four types of RTA have been described:

(a) Type 1 or classical RTA caused by a failure of the distal tubules to excrete hydrogen ions and which is associated with hypokalaemia and also nephrocalcinosis.
(b) Type 2 RTA is due to proximal tubular disease in which a failure to conserve bicarbonate ions occurs, and where there can also be hypokalaemia and Fanconi's syndrome.
(c) Type 3 is a combined proximal and distal tubule defect seen in children.
(d) Type 4 is due to a distal tubular defect and is associated with hyperkalaemia.

Type 1 RTA is associated also with other diseases, such as systemic lupus erythematosus, cirrhosis, medullary sponge kidney, hypercalciuria, primary hyperparathyroidism and drugs such as amphotericin. There is also a familial variety inherited as an autosomal dominant trait. Type 2 can also be inherited, but can also be part of the Fanconi syndrome. It can also occur in vitamin D deficiency, primary hyperparathyroidism, in renal tubular poisoning (such as with heavy metals) or acetazolamide. It may also be a result of multiple myeloma or amyloidosis. The type 4 variety is associated with hypoaldosteronism, such as Addison's disease, and also hyporeninaemia, seen in sickle cell disease, interstitial nephritis and diabetes mellitus. Potassium-sparing diuretics and cyclosporin can also evoke the condition.

3. The medical history points to a diagnosis of type 1 RTA. However, some investigations are useful. Apart from assessing the anion gap in plasma, it is also possible to calculate the anion gap for urine. This is done using the same equation (except with urine concentrations of the analytes) if the urine pH is greater than 6.5, or using the following equation if the urine pH is less than 6.5: (sodium + potassium) urine concentration – chloride urine concentration.

In distal RTA, this gap will be positive because of the low urinary ammonium concentration due to the tubular defect in excreting hydrogen ions. In the presence of a normal anion-gap acidosis, a urinary pH exceeding 5.5, measured on fresh urine with a pH meter, is indicative of RTA. However, this is provided that a urinary tract infection due to urea-splitting organisms, such as *Proteus* has been excluded. Sometimes a severe hypokalaemia can evoke ammonia synthesis and thus lead to a comparatively alkaline urine. In such cases, the potassium deficit should be corrected before urine pH determination.

The short oral ammonium chloride test is said to be the definitive test in distal RTA. This results in a fall in plasma bicarbonate concentration and a diagnosis of distal or type 1 RTA can be made if the urine pH fails to decrease below 5.5. When the ammonium chloride test is contraindicated, such as in liver disease, the calcium chloride test can be used instead. Another alternative diagnostic test is measurement of the urine and blood $PaCO_2$ difference. A value less than 15 mmHg suggests distal RTA.

Proximal RTA is more likely if there is evidence of Fanconi's syndrome, i.e. aminoaciduria, glycosuria, and increased urate and potassium urinary excretion. Unlike type 1 or distal RTA, these patients are still able to produce an acidic urine. The definitive test is the bicarbonate-loading test which is contraindicated in congestive cardiac failure. In a normal individual, bicarbonate does not show in the urine until the plasma bicarbonate concentration exceeds about 26 mmol/l. However, in proximal RTA, the fractional excretion of bicarbonate is more than 15%. The diagnosis of type 4 RTA is helped by noting the hyperkalaemia. Measurement of plasma renin and aldosterone may also be necessary.

Case 44

A 31-year-old electrician attended his general practitioner because of intermittent headaches and dizzy spells, sometimes associated with sweating attacks. He had always been in good health and was not taking any medication. He smoked 10 cigarettes per day and consumed three pints of lager at weekends. On examination, he was found to have a blood pressure of 170/112 standing, and 168/110 lying down. Fundoscopy showed hypertensive changes but no papilloedema.

His pulse was 92 beats/min and the only other significant finding was glycosuria on dipstick testing. The doctor sent blood for biochemical testing and the following results were obtained: sodium 145 mmol/l; potassium 4.5 mmol/l; urea 6.5 mmol/l; creatinine 0.12 mmol/l; random venous plasma glucose 12.4 mmol/l; TSH 1.5 mU/l; fT4 12.4 pmol/l. Upon the basis of these results, the general practitioner had a possible diagnosis in mind and phoned the local consultant chemical pathologist for his advice regarding pertinent biochemical investigations.

Questions

1. What diagnosis did the doctor have in mind?
2. What investigations would help confirm the diagnosis?
3. What endocrine abnormalities can this disorder be associated with?

Answers

1. The general practitioner had a phaeochromocytoma in mind. This diagnosis should always be considered in a patient presenting with these symptoms and hypertension. The hyperglycaemia would be in keeping with this diagnosis and is due to increased catecholamine activity.
2. Phaeochromocytomas are great imitators of many conditions. Although they are potentially curable by surgery, they are also potentially fatal if missed. It is therefore, important, to have a high suspicion of the condition and to use screening tests that are highly sensitive and specific. There has been debate as to the best screening test, with some advocating urinary metanephrines, others urinary 4-hydroxy-3-methoxy mandelic acid (HMMA, but also incorrectly called VMA), and others proposing urinary total free catecholamines (noradrenaline + adrenaline). None of the methods are totally infallible, and some workers suggest using more than one test.
   The decision depends partly upon methodological assay techniques and the likelihood of interfering substances. It has also been suggested that increased excretion of urinary dopamine and homovanillic acid (HVA) are suggestive of the malignant form of phaeochromocytoma. In practice, problems arise in patients in whom catecholamine secretion may be

episodic. In such cases, plasma catecholamine concentrations can be assayed. Other indications for plasma catecholamine determination include borderline elevation of urinary HMMA or metanephrines in patients taking certain catecholamine influencing drugs, e.g beta-blockers, and those patients with renal impairment.

One potential problem is that anxiety can elevate adrenaline levels. In some cases, a pentolinium-suppression test may be useful. Pentolinium is a ganglion-blocking drug and usually suppresses catecholamines in normal subjects. However, autonomous catecholamine release by phaeochromocytomas should not be suppressed. Suppression by clonidine has also been advocated, but this is long-acting and potentially sedative in nature. Once a diagnosis of a phaeochromocytoma has been made, anatomical localization becomes important for surgery. Remember the 'law of 10s' concerning phaeochromocytomas; 10% are malignant, 10% are familial, 10% are bilateral and 10% are extra-adrenal. Scanning by computerized tomography can be useful, as can the radioisotope meta-iodobenzylguanine scan. In some cases, selective venous sampling of catecholamines to help localize the tumour may be necessary, using a catheter passed via the femoral vein into the adrenal veins and the inferior vena cava.

3. Phaeochromocytomas can be associated with the multiple endocrine neoplasia (MEN) syndrome 2, which consists also of medullary carcinoma of the thyroid and parathyroid adenoma. This condition, sometimes known as Sipple's syndrome, can be subgrouped into 2A and 2B, with the latter showing the additional features of a marfanoid appearance and also mucosal neuromas. The MEN 2A syndrome is autosomal-dominant and the gene is located near the centromere of chromosome 10A.

If this syndrome is suspected, near-relatives should be screened for features of the condition. Plasma calcitonin can be used to screen for the syndrome, as elevated levels are associated with medullary carcinoma of the thyroid, being synthesized by the perifollicular 'C' cells. As basal calcitonin plasma concentrations may not always be elevated, the pentagastrin provocative test or calcium infusion can also be used for screening.

Case 45

A three-month-old male child was referred to the paediatricians because of failure to thrive and drowsiness. He had been breast-fed since birth, and was born at term with no complications and by a normal vaginal delivery. He had two sisters aged four and six years who were normal. His mother thought that her mother had lost a baby boy at about six months of age but she was unsure as to the reason. Examination revealed a baby slightly smaller in weight expected for his age. Furthermore, the baby was moderately hypotonic. A number of laboratory investigations were requested, the results of some of which are depicted here: sodium 135 mmol/l; potassium 3.5 mmol/l; chloride 105 mmol/l; bicarbonate 24 mmol/l; urea 0.4 mmol/l; creatinine 0.05 mmol/l. Plasma alanine and glutamine were elevated, while the plasma ammonia concentration was 566 μmol/l. Urine organic acids were normal and there were no ketones detected in the urine.

Questions

1. Suggest a likely diagnosis.
2. What further investigations are necessary to confirm this?
3. What are other causes of hyperammonaemia?

Answers

1. In the face of these results, a urea-cycle disorder should be considered. In an acutely ill child with severe hyperammonaemia, the main differential diagnosis is between an organic acidaemia and a urea-cycle disorder. The absence of a metabolic acidosis and the presence of normal urinary organic acids favours the latter diagnosis, particularly as the plasma urea is low (as in this patient). Interestingly, patients with a urea-cycle disorder tend to have a respiratory alkalosis and also an absence of ketouria.

   The two principle urea-cycle disorders that usually give such a degree of hyperammonaemia are carbamoylphosphate synthetase (CPS) deficiency or ornithine carbomyltransferase (OCT) deficiency. The latter is inherited as an X-linked condition, and thus would fit well with this infant, being male and with a family history of an unexplained male infant death.

The other urea-cycle disorders include N-acetylglutamate synthetase deficiency, argininosuccinate synthetase deficiency, argininosuccinate lyase deficiency, and arginase deficiency. Increases in the plasma and urine of the amino-acids citrulline, argininosuccinic acid and arginine, respectively, are found in the latter three urea-cycle disorders. Plasma ammonia can be almost normal in arginase deficiency depending upon the disorder's severity and diet, whereas concentrations as high as 1500 μmol/l have been described in CPS.

2. A useful biochemical test to distinguish between CPS and OCT is to measure urinary orotic acid, usually by high-performance liquid chromatography or high-voltage electrophoresis. Urinary orotic acid is elevated in OCT but not in CPS. Liver biopsy is useful in finally clinching the enzyme defect when the individual enzymes can be assayed. More recently, DNA probes and molecular biology techniques can be used to screen family members and for prenatal screening.

3. Firstly, it should be realized that hyperammonaemia can often be seen in premature babies and 'ill' neonates reaching concentrations of about 100–200 μmol/l. Care is needed in the collection of samples for plasma ammonia determination as levels up to about 100 μmol/l have been shown in normal healthy neonates within the first three days of life, particularly if capillary blood is used. Thus, venous blood or even arterial blood is to be preferred. Further caution is needed as contaminated collection bottles and old samples can cause spuriously elevated ammonia concentrations.

Apart from the urea-cycle disorders and organic acidurias, other conditions to be excluded include hepatic damage, Reye's syndrome, shock states, sepsis, malignant disease such

Table 24 Some causes of hyperammonaemia

Liver disease
Premature infants
'Ill' neonates, e.g sepsis
High protein intake, sometimes with total parenteral nutrition
Drugs, e.g. sodium valproate
Congenital metabolic defects
• Urea-cycle defects
• Lysine protein intolerance
• Some organic acidurias
• Non-ketotic hyperglycinaemia
• Ornithinaemia and hyperlysinaemia

as leukaemias and the metabolic abnormality of lysinuric protein intolerance (*Table 24*). The antiepileptic drug, valproate, can cause moderate hyperammonaemia, as can total parenteral nutrition.

Case 46

A 16-year-old schoolgirl attended the antenatal clinic claiming to be fourteen weeks' pregnant by her dates. However, physical examination suggested that she was nearer seventeen weeks' pregnant. Her health was otherwise well, with her blood pressure at 100/68. She smoked 10 cigarettes per day. Blood was taken for routine antenatal screening, including a serum alpha-fetoprotein (AFP) test for neural-tube defects. However, after having the blood tests, she walked out of the clinic refusing any more tests. A few days later the results were phoned back to the antenatal clinic; the AFP was 89 KU/l (median being 38 KU/l for seventeen weeks' gestation).

Questions

1. What could be causes of an elevated serum AFP in this patient?
2. What other investigations could be performed?
3. Apart from neural-tube screening, what other antenatal screening role does serum AFP have?

Answers

1. Maternal serum AFP starts to increase from pre-pregnant values from before 10 weeks gestation rising to a maximum at between 30–32 weeks' gestation. One of the main uses of maternal serum AFP determination is to screen for fetal neural-tube defects. It is recommended that blood samples are taken after 16–18 weeks' of gestation and ideally not later than 20–22 weeks. The basis of the test is that, in the event of an open neural tube defect including spina bifida, encephalo-

coele or anencephaly, neural tissue components leak out from the fetus into the amniotic fluid and hence into the maternal circulation.

For her reputed gestational date, this patient's serum AFP is elevated. A common source of error is incorrect gestational dating. Fetal bleeding is another cause of an elevated maternal serum AFP, as are certain rare fetal abnormalities, such as duodenal and oesophageal atresias, renal disease including Potter's syndrome, and ventral wall defects, e.g. gastroschisis or exomphalos. One should also consider fetal Turner's syndrome, fetal death, or threatened abortion. Multiple pregnancy is another explanation; this was the case in this patient who eventually had twins.

2. Unfortunately the patient did not stay long enough for an ultrasound investigation. This can usually show up multiple pregnancies and sometimes also neural tube defects and other congenital abnormalities. If the maternal serum AFP is genuinely elevated for the gestational age and a neural tube defect is suspected, then an amniocentesis can be performed after a confirmatory repeat serum AFP determination. Amniotic AFP can then be assayed and would be expected to be elevated in cases of open neural-tube defects. Another determination that can be made from the amniotic fluid is the level of acetylcholinesterase (AChE), which also derives from the exposed neural tissue. The assay for amniotic AChE is usually made by polyacrylamide gel electrophoresis and shows the presence of non-specific esterases but also a fast neural tube defect band.

3. Maternal serum AFP can also be used as part of the screen for fetal Down's syndrome (trisomy 21) when there is an association with low concentrations of AFP. The possible explanation is that in Down's syndrome the fetal liver produces less AFP. Maternal serum AFP concentrations should be corrected for maternal age and weight and it should also be remembered that levels can be lower in maternal diabetes mellitus. Other assays performed on maternal serum as part of the Down's syndrome screen include human chorionic gonadotrophin (beta-HCG) which tends to be elevated in the syndrome, and unconjugated oestriol which tends to be decreased. There is presently some debate as to whether beta-HCG or its free beta subunit are the best parameter to measure. In suspected cases, amniocentesis is again necessary when samples are taken for karotyping of fetal cultured cells.

Case 47

A 31-year-old staff nurse was seen in the general medical clinic because of dizzy spells, sweating episodes and weakness. These attacks had been worsening over the preceding five months. Her health had been otherwise good and she was not taking any medication except the oral contraceptive pill. She did not like alcohol and was a non-smoker. She had no social problems nor any depressive symptoms. On direct questioning, she complained of nocturnal hunger. Physical examination was unremarkable and her blood pressure was 120/70. A resting ECG was normal. The attending physician wondered whether hypogly-caemia was causing her symptoms and he arranged for her hospital admission and a prolonged fast. Within 18 hours of the fast, she felt dizzy, started to sweat and felt weak. A blood glucose measured at this time showed a venous plasma glucose of 1.8 mmol/l. Blood was also taken for insulin determination which was shown to be 184 pmol/l. She was given intravenous glucose which resulted in prompt improvement of her symptoms.

Questions

1. What is a possible diagnosis?
2. What is Whipple's triad?
3. Discuss any further investigations that may be indicated.
4. What other causes of hypoglycaemia can be encountered in patients?.

Answers

1. Insulinoma is likely upon the basis of symptomatic hypogly-caemia in the presence of inappropriately high plasma insulin levels. An insulinoma is usually a tumour of the pancreatic islet cells and can be a feature of the multiple endocrine neoplasia syndrome, e.g. MEN1. In this latter condition, an insulinoma can be associated with adenomas of the anterior pituitary gland and also the parathyroid.
2. The prolonged fast in this patient has demonstrated Whipple's triad, i.e. symptoms suggestive of hypoglycaemia during the fasting, confirmation of hypoglycaemia by blood analysis, and

reversal of symptoms upon administration of glucose. These features together are strongly suggestive of an insulinoma.

3. The prolonged fast is useful in making the diagnosis of insulinoma. However, close medical supervision is needed because of the possible need to give glucose. Factitious hypoglycaemia, due to insulin self-administration, should be excluded by also measuring serum insulin C-peptide at the time of hypoglycaemia. This peptide should be high in patients with an insulinoma, i.e. an endogenous source of insulin. In a patient surreptitiously injecting exogenous insulin, serum C-peptide levels would be unlikely to be detected, i.e the endogenous production would be suppressed. Patients who secretly take a hypoglycaemic-evoking drug, e.g a sulphonylurea, are difficult to uncover despite serum C-peptide determinations. In these cases, serum drug assays are useful.

Other tests to investigate insulinoma have included the fish insulin suppression test and assays of serum proinsulin. If MEN1 is suspected, other features of the syndrome should be looked for, such as hyperparathyroidism and adenomas of the anterior pituitary. Once a diagnosis of insulinoma has been made, localization of the tumour is necessary. Many techniques are available, including computerized tomography scans, ultrasound, and angiography of the coeliac axis. Some units prefer selective venous sampling of veins draining the pancreatic area; a recent modification is to sample for insulin from these venous sites after calcium infusion.

4. Hypoglycaemia is usually defined as a plasma venous plasma glucose less than 2.8 mmol/l. There are many causes of hypoglycaemia apart from those already mentioned (*Table 25*). Starvation and alcohol consumption are well described, as is the use of drugs such as salicylates and monoamine oxidase inhibitors in relatively high dosage. Endocrine causes include hypopituitarism and adrenal insufficiency. Severe liver disease and also tumours, such as neuroblastomas or retroperitoneal sarcomas, are also causes. Inherited abnormalities include glycogen storage disease, galactosaemia and fructose and leucine sensitivity. Remember also iatrogenic causes of hypoglycaemia, such as treated diabetics on either insulin or hypoglycaemic drugs, and in some patients postgastrectomy. Reactive hypoglycaemia has also been described in some individuals in response to oral glucose intake.

115

Table 25 Some causes of hypoglycaemia

Excess of insulin or hypoglycaemic drug
- Neonatal forms
- Prematurity
- Childhood forms
- Leucine sensitivity
- Glycogen storage disease
- Galactosaemia

Reactive types
- Post-gastrectomy
- In response to ethanol, fructose or galactose

Fasting types
- Insulinoma
- 'Hungry tumours', e.g retroperitoneal sarcoma
- Severe hepatic disease
- Adrenal insufficiency
- Hypopituitarism

Functional form
- Physiological
- Prolonged fasting
- Strenuous exercise
- Pregnancy

Case 48

A four-year-old boy was admitted under the care of the paediatricians for chemotherapy treatment of an acute lymphoblastic leukaemia. He had initially presented a few weeks earlier with spontaneous bruising, lethargy and recurrent throat infections. A course of chemotherapy was proposed consisting of vincristine, prednisolone, asparaginase and adriamycin. Prior to chemotherapy, he was given oral allopurinol. Routine biochemistry and also haematology tests were performed each day after his chemotherapy course. The results of the blood biochemistry tests performed two days after the initiation of chemotherapy were: sodium 136 mmol/l; potassium 5.6 mmol/l; urea 7.8 mmol/l; creatinine 0.13 mmol/l; calcium 2.10 mmol/l; phosphate 3.40 mmol/l; albumin 35 g/l; urate 0.54 mmol/l.

Questions

1. Comment upon the plasma urate result.
2. Give a possible explanation for the potassium and phosphate results in this patient.
3. What causes hyperuricaemia in hospital patients?

Answers

1. The plasma urate is moderately raised. The rapid growth of dividing tumour cells and consequently the elevated nucleic acid turnover result in increased purine metabolism and hyperuricaemia. Not only can the raised plasma urate be attributed to overproduction, but the chemotherapy regime will destroy tumour cells and in so doing exacerbate the hyperuricaemia as urate is released from damaged cells. Although this has been described for a number of tumours, lymphoblastic malignancies are said to show this feature readily because of their fast lysis rate. It is interesting that elevated plasma urate concentrations occurred in this patient despite prophylactic treatment with the xanthine oxidase inhibitor, allopurinol. It is important to monitor plasma urate concentrations in patients with malignant disease, particularly if on chemotherapy, as high levels of urate can cause an obstructive nephropathy by precipitating in the collecting ducts and distal tubules. Thus bear in mind that urate is filtered at the renal glomerulus, then reabsorbed at the proximal tubules and resecreted in the distal tubules. The renal function tests of this patient do not show major impairment. Sometimes plasma urate concentrations can reach very high levels, and may present with nausea, anorexia and lethargy and even gout or renal colic.
2. Note also that this patient has hyperkalaemia and hyperphosphataemia. The reference range for plasma phosphate in a child of this age is about 1.2–1.9 mmol/l, i.e. it is higher than that for adults. Although these conditions can be elevated in renal failure, the patient's renal function tests do not suggest this. The explanation can also be attributed to the chemotherapy and tumour cell breakdown as both potassium and phosphate are intracellular ions that are released from the cells upon lysis. Collectively, the features of hyperkalaemia, hyperphosphataemia and hyperuricaemia in patients under-

going tumour treatment have been termed the 'tumour lysis syndrome'. In severe cases, lifethreatening hyperkalaemia can result, and severe hyperphosphataemia can result in hypocalcaemia.

3. It is useful to divide hyperuricaemia into primary and secondary causes (*Table 26*). Rare causes of primary hyperuricaemia include glucose-6-phosphatase deficiency (Von Gierke's disease), and also the Lesch-Nyhan syndrome, due to a deficiency of the enzyme hypoxanthine guanine phosphoribosyl transferase. Hyperuricaemia can also be a feature of Down's syndrome. Idiopathic gout is also thought to be a primary abnormality in which about 80% of individuals show enhanced urate production while about 20% show reduced renal excretion.

Table 26 Some causes of hyperuricaemia

Primary causes	Idiopathic gout or hyperuricaemia
	Von Gierke's disease (deficiency of glucose-6-phosphate)
	Lesch-Nyhan syndrome
	Sometimes in Down's syndrome
Secondary causes	Acute or chronic renal failure
	Drugs, e.g thiazides, low-dose salicylate, pyrazinamide
	Some tumours, myeloproliferative disease
	Severe tissue breakdown
	Lead poisoning
	Association with hypertriglyceridaemia/hypertension and Insulin resistance
	Sometimes in acidotic conditions
	Pregnancy-related hypertension

The secondary causes can be subclassified into those resulting from increased urate production and those due to impaired renal excretion of urate. In the case of the former, increased nucleic acid turnover has already been discussed in the context of tumours, but myeloproliferative disease and severe psoriasis can also result in hyperuricaemia. The latter group consists of drugs that reduce renal tubular secretion of urate, such as low-dose salicylates, pyrazinamide, frusemide and thiazide diuretics, as well as renal disease, including both acute and chronic renal failure, and also nephrotoxicity due to lead poisoning. Both ketone bodies and lactic acid can inhibit renal tubule secretion of urate leading to hyperuricaemia.

Some individuals are particularly prone to dietary elevation of urate, as a result of either high ethanol consumption or high meat consumption, i.e purine-rich diets. Hyperuricaemia can be a feature of pregnancy-related hypertension and also hypertriglyceridaemia.

Case 49

A 61-year-old Asian warehouseman attended his general practitioner because of polydipsia that had started about three months previously. Otherwise, he had no other complaints, although he was being treated for hypertension with a calcium antagonist. He had undergone two inguinal hernia operations three and five years ago. Furthermore, he smoked 15 cigarettes per day, but did not drink alcohol. In his family history, he thought that his father had suffered from 'sugar in his urine'. On physical examination he had a blood pressure of 156/94 and was obviously overweight with a body mass index of 28.6. There was nothing else of note upon examination. The practice nurse tested the patient's urine and found a trace of glucose but no ketones. The general practitioner suspected diabetes mellitus and arranged for an oral glucose tolerance test and a fasting lipid screen at the local hospital. The following results were sent back to the doctor a few days later: cholesterol 6.6 mmol/l; triglyceride 5.3 mmol/l; HDL-cholesterol 0.80 mmol/l. Oral glucose tolerance tests results for venous whole blood;(75g of anhydrous glucose given)

- 0   hour   6.9 mmol/l
- ½   hour   13.1 mmol/l
- 1   hour   12.0 mmol/l
- 2   hour   11.9 mmol/l

Questions

1. Does the patient have diabetes mellitus?
2. Comment upon the biochemical results and also the findings of clinical examination.

3. Give a list of causes of hyperglycaemia that can be encountered in patients.

Answers

1. Based upon the glucose tolerance test results and also the symptoms experienced by the patient, diabetes mellitus is the correct diagnosis. It is important to understand the diagnostic criteria proposed by the WHO for the oral glucose tolerance test. Firstly, the patient should be properly prepared for the test, being previously on a normal diet containing more than 150 g of carbohydrate for three days prior to the test. The patient should fast for between 10–16 hours, the test should be performed in the morning, and the patient should not smoke or exercise during the test. The patient should only drink water while fasting for the test and should not be taking any drugs known to interfere with glucose metabolism. Glucose should be assayed by a laboratory glucose enzymatic assay, and it should be stated whether venous, capillary, or whole blood was used. The WHO diagnostic criteria for diabetes mellitus, using venous whole blood is a fasting blood glucose of greater than or equal to 6.7 mmol/l and/or a two-hour post-oral blood glucose of equal to, or greater than, 10 mmol/l. These criteria differ according to whether venous or whole blood are used, since venous plasma glucose is usually about 15% higher than venous whole blood values. Thus, the plasma glucose criteria for venous plasma are 7.8 mmol/l fasting and 11.1 mmol/l for the two hour-sample.

The oral glucose tolerance test is undoubtedly an over-prescribed test. The WHO 1985 report proposed that, as an initial screen, a random venous plasma glucose greater than 11.1 mmol/l was diagnostic for diabetes mellitus. However, they omitted a fasting value due to the problems of ensuring patient compliance. Nevertheless, in equivocal cases, the oral glucose tolerance test is needed. It is also worth pointing out the condition of impaired glucose tolerance. Based upon a venous whole blood sample, a fasting value of less than 6.7 mmol/l and a two-hour post-oral glucose of between 6.7–10.0 mmol/l show impaired glucose tolerance. This condition is of relevance in pregnancy (gestational diabetes mellitus). It also carries the risk of developing frank diabetes mellitus as well as putting the individual at risk of cardiovascular disease.

2. This patient, who was later diagnosed as having non-insulin dependent diabetes mellitus (NIDDM) (also known as type 2 or late-onset diabetes mellitus), is overweight and has hypertension. In contrast, type 1 diabetes mellitus is the insulin-dependent variety and tends to occur in younger subjects. Furthermore, this man has a dyslipidaemia with elevated fasting triglycerides and a low HDL-cholesterol. There has been much recent interest in the aggregation of these features in individuals, and evidence suggests that these are part of the insulin-resistance syndrome (syndrome X or Reaven's syndrome). These patients are at risk of cardiovascular disease. Such individuals also have a tendency to central obesity as judged by hip:waist ratios, and there is also a racial difference with the syndrome being well-described in some Asians.

3. Hyperglycaemia is also a feature of malnutrition-related diabetes mellitus, which has been subgrouped into protein-deficient pancreatic diabetes and fibrocalculous pancreatic diabetes. Other types of diabetes are associated with pancreatic disease and endocrinal causes, such as Cushing's syndrome, acromegaly, glucagonoma and phaeochromocytoma. Drugs should also be remembered, including glucocorticoids, thiazides and phenothiazines. There is also an association with genetic syndromes, including Down's and Turner's syndromes, congenital lipodystrophy and ataxia telangiectasia (*Table 27*).

Table 27 Some causes of hyperglycaemia

Insulin-dependent diabetes mellitus type 1
Non-insulin dependent diabetes mellitus (obese or non-obese) type 2
Malnutrition-related diabetes mellitus
Impaired glucose tolerance
Gestational diabetes mellitus

Other forms of diabetes mellitus
Associated with genetic syndromes, e.g. Turner's syndrome
Some of the glycogen-storage diseases, ataxia telangiectasia, DIDMOAD
Diseases of the pancreas
Endocrine causes, e.g. Cushing's syndrome, phaeochromocytoma, acromegaly
Drugs, e.g. thiazides, glucocorticoids
Sometimes with peritoneal dialysis

Case 50

A 15-year-old schoolboy had been referred to the neurology out-patients because of a slowly progressing dysarthria and weakness in his legs. He had been getting less well over the last year and had missed a lot of time from school because of headaches and tiredness. Prior to this, he had been well and enjoyed school, although he was finding it difficult to keep up with his classwork. He was not taking any medication. He had one sister who was well, but his mother told the doctor that her sister had died in her thirties from a 'liver problem'. A number of investigations were performed, including biochemistry blood tests. The results are presented here: sodium 143 mmol/l; potassium 3.4 mmol/l; urea 5.7 mmol/l; creatinine 0.11 mmol/l; calcium 2.22 mmol/l; phosphate 0.78 mmol/l; urate 0.05 mmol/l; albumin 35 g/l; alanine transaminase 94 U/l; alkaline phosphatase 334 U/l; bilirubin 9 μmol/l; random venous plasma glucose 4.5 mmol/l. Analysis of a 24-hour urine collection was reported as showing moderate generalized aminoaciduria.

Questions

1. Suggest a likely diagnosis.
2. What investigations could you perform to confirm this?
3. Apart from the liver function tests, comment upon the abnormal biochemistry results.
4. What causes of hypouricaemia can be found in hospital patients?

Answers

1. In the face of abnormal liver function tests, neurological manifestations, a family history of a liver disorder and aminoaciduria, one should consider Wilson's disease. This is a rare autosomal condition with a disease prevalence of about 1 in 30 000. The metabolic defect results in an accumulation of copper in the tissues, notably the liver and brain. Untreated death often results in the third to fourth decade of life due to cirrhosis or extrapyramidal degeneration. Other features of the disease include haemolytic anaemia, gall-stones, osteoporosis and renal tubular defects.

2. Slit-lamp examination of the eyes may show Kayser-Fleischer rings, the result of pigment deposition in the medial and lateral aspects of the cornea. This physical sign would strongly substantiate a diagnosis of Wilson's disease, but is not pathogonomic as it may be a feature of other hepatic disease, such as primary biliary cirrhosis. In view of this, biochemical tests are essential in making a diagnosis.

The actual metabolic defect in Wilson's disease is thought to be due to an abnormality in the incorporation of copper into copper-binding proteins in the liver. The main copper-binding protein is caeruloplasmin and serum concentrations are often low in Wilson's disease as is the serum total copper concentration. However, sometimes serum caeruloplasmin and total copper concentrations are normal in Wilson's disease, and alternative tests become necessary. An elevated free serum copper, however, has been shown to be almost 100% specific and sensitive for this disorder and is probably the screening test of choice. Indeed, it is the free serum copper (also known as noncaeruloplasmin serum copper) which is toxic in Wilson's disease. This can be quantitated by the following equation: free serum copper = total serum copper − serum caeruloplasmin bound copper. In this context, if is useful to know that one mg of caeruloplasmin binds 0.047 μmol of copper. Some workers also measure urinary copper excretion which is frequently elevated in Wilson's disease and usually exceeds 1 μmol/24 hours. It used to be taught that determining liver copper deposition by a liver biopsy was the best way to make the diagnosis of Wilson's disease, with more than 3.9 μmol/l of copper per gram dry weight of liver being indicative. However, other hepatic disorders can result in elevated hepatic copper levels, such as primary biliary cirrhosis.

3. This patient has hypokalaemia, hypophosphataemia, hypouricaemia and a generalized aminoaciduria. These are indicative of Fanconi's syndrome, a generalized defect of the renal tubules, where there is tubular leakage of potassium, phosphate, urate and amino acids. Fanconi's syndrome can be either a primary inherited abnormality or secondary to renal tubule damage. Glycosuria can also be a feature. Fanconi's syndrome is a well-described feature of Wilson's disease, presumably due to the effect of copper toxicity upon the renal tubules.

Aminoaciduria can be classified into two groups. Generalized renal aminoaciduria is seen in this patient, but overflow aminoaciduria can also occur. This is the result of increased urinary excretion of amino-acid(s) due to increased plasma amino-acid concentrations. The latter situation can be observed in phenylketonuria or homocystinuria, or as a result of hepatic disease or increased tissue breakdown. Apart from Wilson's disease, renal aminoaciduria can also result from renal damage due to heavy metals, oculo-cerebro-renal syndrome, galactosaemia, cystinosis and hereditary fructose intolerance.

4. Hypouricaemia is rare. It can either be due to increased urinary excretion, as in Fanconi's syndrome, or be caused by uricosuric drugs, such as probenecid or high-dose salicylate. An increased urinary excretion of urate also occurs in early pregnancy, diabetes mellitus and in the syndrome of inappropriate antidiuretic hormone (SIADH). Decreased urate production is another cause of hypouricaemia as it is seen after allopurinol treatment for gout. Allopurinol is a xanthine oxidase inhibitor. A rare deficiency of xanthine oxidase has also been described resulting in hypouricaemia and xanthinuria (*Table 28*).

Table 28 Some causes of hypouricaemia

Urate lowering drugs, e.g. allopurinol, probenecid
Fanconi's syndrome
Myeloma
Wilson's disease
Syndrome of inappropriate ADH
Genetic, e.g deficiency of nucleoside phosphorylase, xanthine oxidase or adenosine deaminase

Case 51

A 66-year-old retired toolmaker attended casualty because of increasing dyspnoea. He had suffered from chronic obstructive airways disease (COAD) for about 10 years. He smoked 30 cigarettes per day, having refused to stop the habit, and drank five pints of beer per week. His usual medication was a salbutamol inhaler and he took slow-release theophylline tablets orally. However, he admitted to increasing his dose of the latter over the last few days because of his breathlessness. Over the last two days, he had become increasingly more breathless with the production of copious green phlegm. In his past medical history, he had an attack of shingles five years ago and an inguinal hernia operation 10 years ago. On examination, he was clearly distressed and looked centrally cyanosed. His heart rate was 98/min, respiratory rate 24/min and his blood pressure 146/90. He also had bilateral pitting oedema of his ankles and distended neck veins. His chest showed variable wheezes and crackles with a prolonged expiratory phase. The attending medical officer also noted he had a slight hand tremor. A number of emergency blood tests were sent to the laboratory: sodium 138 mmol/l; potassium 3.6 mmol/l; chloride 90 mmol/l; bicarbonate 39 mmol/l; urea 8.7 mmol/l; creatinine 0.12 mmol/l; theophylline 30 mg/l. Arterial blood gases were also sent a little later, with the following results: pH 7.30; $PaCO_2$ 70 mmHg; PaO_2 53 mmHg.

Questions

1. What is the acid/base disturbance?
2. Comment upon the theophylline plasma concentration.
3. What other conditions can give rise to this type of acid/base abnormality?

Answers

1. This patient shows a respiratory acidosis. Note that the blood pH shows an acidaemia and the $PaCO_2$ is elevated. The compensation mechanism for this condition involves the kidneys which increase their tubular secretion of hydrogen ions as well as increasing their reabsorption and generation of bicarbonate. This latter mechanism explains the elevated plasma bicarbonate concentration in this patient. This observation is also a clue that the respiratory problem has occurred over a relatively long time (days rather than hours) as an attempt at renal compensation has taken place. Chronic lung disease is a well-established cause of a respiratory acidosis, where there is impaired carbon dioxide excretion by the lungs.

The danger for these patients is the possibility of respiratory failure. This is usually defined as an arterial PaO_2 of less than 60 mmHg with or without a $PaCO_2$ of greater than 50 mmHg. Respiratory failure itself can be subclassified into three broad groups:

(a) Hypoxaemic failure which manifests as a low PaO_2 with a normal or even low $PaCO_2$. This is usually the result of alveolar mismatching of ventilation and perfusion.
(b) So-called ventilatory failure in which there is a decreased PaO_2 and an elevated $PaCO_2$. The predominant defect here is impairment of alveolar ventilation.
(c) A mixed respiratory failure which is a combination of the previous two conditions.

Another biochemical fact worth remembering when it comes to treating such a patient is the danger of carbon dioxide narcosis as a result of inadequately controlled oxygen therapy. Patients with a chronically elevated $PaCO_2$ depend upon a hypoxic drive to stimulate their respiration. If there is a brisk, unmonitored increase in their PaO_2, this hypoxic drive can become blunted and further depress respiration leading to further carbon dioxide retention.

2. The patient had admitted to increasing his oral aminophylline medication and the medical officer had noticed the patient's tremor, which can be a sign of theophylline toxicity. The plasma theophylline concentration is high in this patient, with the therapeutic range usually quoted at between 5–20 mg/l. Toxic effects of theophylline include headaches, nausea, tremor, vomiting, cardiac arrhythmias and convulsions. It can thus be worth measuring plasma theophylline levels in patients suspected of showing toxic symptoms or signs. Some of the theophylline oral preparations are slow-release and thus it may be useful to repeat plasma levels about four hours after a previously elevated result to see whether these values are increasing due to continuing drug absorption.

3. Other causes of a respiratory acidosis (*Table 29*) include intrinsic lung disease, such as asthma, chronic bronchitis and emphysema. Obstruction of the bronchial airways, e.g. due to tumours or foreign body, should also be considered, as should neuromuscular disorders including the Guillain-Barré syndrome and poliomyelitis. Respiratory depressants are another cause, particularly of note are narcotics, anaesthetics and sedatives.

Table 29 Some causes of a respiratory acidosis

Intrinsic lung disease	Asthma
	Emphysema
	Bronchitis
	Pneumonia
	Fibrosing alveolitis
Respiratory centre depression	Infections
	Cerebrovascular accidents
	Tumours
	Some sedative drugs
Ventilation/perfusion defects	Pulmonary emboli
Neuromuscular defects of respiratory muscles	Poliomyelitis
	Guillain-Barré syndrome
Primary alveolar hypoventilation (Pickwickian syndrome)	
'Shock lung' syndrome	

Case 52

A 72-year-old retired builder attended his general practitioner because of pain in his left leg. This was localized to his femur and was aching in nature and worse at night. He had started to limp over the last four months. He was not on any medication and was a non-smoker. His health previously had been excellent and this was the first time that he had visited a doctor for 30 years. However, he did volunteer that he had become more deaf over the last year. On physical examination, he was tender over his left femur and there was bowing of his lower limbs. However, there was no limb shortening and the rest of the examination was normal with no signs of cardiac failure or disorders of his nervous system. The general practitioner arranged for X-rays of his lower limbs and also a blood test by the local clinical chemistry laboratory. The results of the chemistry tests are shown here: calcium 2.45 mmol/l; phosphate 0.95 mmol/l; albumin 40 g/l; alkaline phosphatase 899 U/l. The X-rays were reported as showing osteosclerotic areas with expansion of bone and loss of the normal bone trabecular pattern.

Questions

1. Suggest a likely diagnosis.
2. What are the predominant alkaline phosphatase isoenzymes found in human serum?
3. At the other extreme of age, markedly elevated serum alkaline phosphatase has been described in apparently healthy infants. What is this condition?

Answers

1. The X-ray findings, symptoms of bone pain and also deafness, lower limb bowing and deformity and a very elevated serum alkaline phosphatase activity suggest Paget's disease.

   The cause of this bone disease is not known, but the features include increased turnover of bone collagen and mineral content, as a result of increased osteoclastic resorption, and increased new bone formation. The new bone is laid down in a disorganized fashion. Complications include vertebral compression, high output cardiac failure, skull enlargement, and the trapping of nerves by foraminal encroachment. The latter feature presumably explains the nerve deafness that this patient had experienced. A rare complication includes the development of osteosarcoma associated with sudden increase in bone pain and a large increase in serum alkaline phosphatase.

   Other useful investigations include bone scanning and also urinary hydroxyproline excretion (which when elevated reflects increased bone resorption). Future developments in bone-specific acid phosphatase and alkaline phosphatase assays may be of further use, as may the assay of serum osteo-calcin (a bone protein) and also collagen cross-links (reflecting new bone formation). Remember that hypercalcaemia is not usually a feature of Paget's disease unless the patient becomes immobilized.

2. In the presence of the clinical findings and X-ray appearances, one assumes that the elevated alkaline phosphatase is predominantly due to the bone isoenzyme. However, the other predominant serum alkaline phosphatase isoenzymes include liver, intestine and placenta. These can be distinguished by electrophoretic or immunological techniques, differential chemical inhibition or heat inactivation, or urea denaturation.

Two additional isoenzymes are sometimes seen in malignancies, and can be used as tumour markers. These are similar to the placental isoenzyme in that they are relatively heat-resistant. These are the so-called Nagao (sensitive to L-leucine inhibition) and Regan isoenzymes. A renal isoenzyme has also been shown and a PA variety sometimes seen in patients with pancreatic carcinoma. This list is not complete as other tissues can produce the enzyme.

3. Although serum alkaline phosphatase is elevated in infancy due to the rapid bone growth of development, markedly elevated levels (about 20–30x upper reference limit) have been described in apparently normal children. This finding has been termed transient hyperphosphataemia of infancy. This may last for several months and the children tend to be younger than two years of age. There is an apparent absence of bone or liver disease, although it is recommended that the children are regularly followed-up. There is debate as to the nature of the alkaline phosphatase isoenzyme with some workers suggesting that it is of bone origin while others propose that it is a variant isoenzyme.

Case 53

A 20-year-old labourer had been referred to the rheumatologists because of arthralgia and Raynaud's syndrome. His symptoms had come on over the last two years when he had started his labouring work and he had noticed that the symptoms were far worse in the winter months. On closer questioning it was found that these symptoms were associated with a purpuric skin rash and occasionally slight ulceration of his fingers. He also mentioned an intense pain in his finger tips, nose and ears when labouring in the cold.

His health otherwise was good with no hospital admissions, apart from breaking his nose in a game of football. He was not taking any medication. He smoked 20 cigarettes per day and drank 10 units of beer per week. He had no idea of any family illnesses as he had run away from home in his teens and had never been close to his parents. Physical examination was unremarkable apart from a slight generalized purpuric rash.

Some initial blood tests were performed and the following results obtained: haemoglobin 14.5 g/dl; white cells 5.6 × 10⁹/l; platelets 178 × 10⁹/l; rheumatoid factor and also antinuclear factor were negative, as were antibodies to double stranded DNA; serum complement C3 was 0.55 g/l (0.80–1.70) and C4 0.11 g/l (0.20–0.70); sodium 144 mmol/l; potassium 4.2 mmol/l; urea 5.6 mmol/l; creatinine 0.09 mmol/l; bilirubin 6 umol/l; alanine transaminase 21 U/l; alkaline phosphatase 121 U/l; random venous plasma glucose 4.2 mmol/l; calcium 2.41 mmol/l; phosphate 0.89 mmol/l; albumin 42 g/l; total protein 72 g/l.

Questions

1. What would be a possible explanation for this man's symptoms?
2. Describe investigations that could be performed to help make a diagnosis.
3. What are some causes for decreased serum C3 and C4 levels?.

Answers

1. The symptoms of arthralgia, purpuric skin rash, Raynaud's syndrome and painful extremities in the cold would suggest the diagnosis of a cryoproteinaemia. This is due to proteins that precipitate or gel upon plasma or serum cooling but which usually redissolve on rewarming to 37°C.

   There are four main groups of cryoprotein. About two-thirds of cases are due to mixed cryoglobulins. These consist of immune complexes which are often polyclonal antibodies against IgG or DNA. These complexes can fix fibrinogen and complement, which can result in synovitis, vasculitis, and even glomerulonephritis and renal failure. A monoclonal cryoglobulin has also been described which in most cases is related to a malignant immunocytoma. Also described is an abnormal form of fibrinogen, called cryofibrinogen, that precipitates only in plasma rather than serum. Finally, cold agglutinins have been found that reversibly agglutinate red cells in the cold, resulting not only in Raynaud's syndrome but also a haemolytic anaemia. In some cases, this is a transient phenomenon being secondary to an infection such as mycoplasma when the agglutinins are often polyclonal IgM.

Cryoproteins can be a feature of malignant disease, infections, autoimmune disorders or liver disease. This patient was found to have none of these conditions. After extensive investigation, it was concluded that he had essential cryoglobulinaemia.

2. Cryoglobulins slowly come out of solution when the plasma or serum is cooled to below body temperature, usually to form a precipitate or gel. On rewarming, these go back into solution. Blood should be collected warm and quickly taken to the laboratory. The sample is then separated to produce plasma or serum in a warm centrifuge and then aliquoted into three portions – one at 37°C, one at room temperature and one at 4°C. The significance of cryoglobulins at 4°C is not clear as obviously this temperature *in vivo* is not attainable during life. If a cryoprecipitate occurs, then the immunoglobulin total content can be quantitated both in the cold supernatant serum and also the body temperature serum and the amount of cryoglobulin quantitated by difference. Monoclonal cryoglobulins can be similarly observed and serum electrophoresis performed on the cold and warm samples followed by immunofixation and staining to quantitate and type the cryoprotein. Cryofibrinogen can also be determined by collecting both a serum and a plasma (oxalate or EDTA) sample. A precipitate observed in the cold which redissolves on warming in the latter, but not in the serum sample, suggests cryofibrinogen.

3. Low complement concentrations suggest either a decreased synthesis or an increased consumption. The former has been observed in severe liver disease but also as a congenital disorder due to structural gene defects. Individuals heterozygous for C4 sometimes also have insulin-dependent diabetes mellitus or systemic lupus erythematosus. An increased complement consumption may be the consequence of antigen-antibody complex formation either as a result of autoimmune disease or infection. If serum C3 is normal, but C4 is low, this could suggest C1 esterase inhibitor deficiency. Conversely, a low serum C3 and normal C4 suggests activation of the alternative pathway due perhaps to a microorganism infection or endotoxin. Remember also that, as a result of the acute phase reaction, serum complement concentrations rise.

Case 54

A 47-year-old lorry driver attended the gastroenterology department because of prolonged diarrhoea which had persisted on and off for about three weeks. There was no blood in his stools but the diarrhoea persisted even when he had tried to fast and was also associated with abdominal discomfort. The stools were watery in nature and not white and did not float in the toilet pan. He also felt flushed at varying times during the day which reminded him of eating spicy foods and which was worsened by drinking alcohol. Furthermore, he thought that he was getting progressively more breathless, particularly on walking up stairs. He was on no medication apart from antidiarrhoeal agents but he did smoke 15 cigarettes a day. He had stopped drinking alcohol since the diarrhoea had started. On examination he looked as if he had lost some body weight. His blood pressure was 146/86 and a systolic cardiac murmur was detected. Examination of his abdomen showed slight distension, but there was otherwise little of note. Rectal examination was normal. A number of gastrointestinal investigations were requested, but then the consultant thought of an explanation for the symptoms. He asked the patient to collect a 24-hour urine sample and take it to the clinical chemistry department.

Questions

1. What diagnosis had the doctor in mind and what investigation was the urine test most likely to be for?
2. What would be a differential diagnosis of the patient's diarrhoea?
3. What other biochemical investigations are of use in investigating patients with diarrhoea?

Answers

1. The doctor felt that carcinoid syndrome was likely and ordered a urinary 5-hydroxyindole acetic acid (5-HIAA) determination. The result came back as 435 µmol/l. This syndrome arises from a tumour of the argentaffin cells, which can arise commonly in the ileocaecal region but also in the lung and

other organs. These tumours secrete large amounts of 5-hydroxytryptamine (5-HT) which is normally metabolized in the liver to various products including 5-HIAA. However, in the event of liver metastasis, the tumour secretions can bypass the portal circulation giving rise to systemic side-effects. These include flushing, diarrhoea, right-sided heart lesions, including pulmonary stenosis, and niacin deficiency resulting in a pellagra-like syndrome. Some tumours, usually of hind-gut origin, may not convert 5-HT to 5-HIAA. If the diagnosis is suspected, but urine concentrations of 5-HIAA are not grossly elevated, then plasma 5-HT assay may be useful. Furthermore, some carcinoid tumours can also secrete ectopic hormones, such as ACTH, giving rise to Cushing's syndrome.

2. Broadly speaking, diarrhoea can be divided into secretory diarrhoea or osmotic diarrhoea. The distinction is not always so clear-cut, but generally the former gives large stool volumes, perhaps more than 1 litre per day due to secretion from the gastrointestinal tract. Conversely, osmotic diarrhoea is often due to ingested solutes which are osmotically active but are not absorbed by the gut and can be seen also in malabsorption states. It is frequently improved by fasting and the stool volume is not as extensive as in the secretory form.

Carcinoid syndrome is one of the secretory diarrhoeas. These can also be the result of increased gastrin secretion, as in Zollinger-Ellison syndrome, increased calcitonin secretion seen in medullary carcinoma of the thyroid, or in the Verner-Morrison syndrome also called the WDHA syndrome (watery diarrhoea, hypokalaemia and achlorhydria) due to a vipoma-secreting vasoactive intestinal polypeptide (VIP). Other causes of secretory diarrhoea include damage to the intestinal mucosa, as in inflammatory bowel disease, bowel infections and bacterial toxins and chronic purgative abuse. Osmotic diarrhoea can be seen in malabsorption states, chloride diarrhoea, osmotic purgative abuse, e.g. magnesium salts and also lactase deficiency.

3. Stools can be cultured and toxins looked for when the cause of the diarrhoea is sought. The distinction between osmotic and secretory diarrhoea can be made by measuring stool osmolality and also the predominant osmotically active cations, namely sodium and potassium. A calculated stool osmolality can be obtained from the following formula; 2X (sodium + potassium stool concentration). The difference between the measured stool osmolality and that calculated is greater than

20 mmol/l in osmotic diarrhoea, i.e there is a significant stool osmolality gap.

In the case of suspected magnesium laxative abuse, magnesium can also be measured in the stool and the gap would thus be expected to be elevated. Other laxatives can also be assayed in urine or stools. In the case of disaccharidase deficiency, reducing sugars are found in the stool, i.e lactose, galactose or glucose, and the stool pH is acidic and usually less than 6. If a secretory diarrhoea is suspected due to excess gut hormone secretion, e.g VIP or gastrin, then these should be measured in fasting blood samples. Sometimes it is necessary to do this on more than one occasion.

The study of malabsorption states is complex and biochemical tests are only part of the investigations required. Radiological imaging techniques, endoscopy and the use of the Crosby capsule to obtain histological material are often more useful. Biochemical tests for pancreatic malabsorption states are covered in another case in this book (p. 71) and would include possibly faecal fat analysis and intubation and tubeless studies. The biochemical diagnosis of jejunal malabsorption can sometimes be aided by faecal fats, a xylose tolerance test, and a red-cell folate determination, whereas ileal malabsorption can be biochemically investigated by the determination of ^{14}C in the stools and $^{14}CO_2$ in the breath after giving radiolabelled glycocholic acid, i.e the bile acid breath test. The Schilling test and faecal fat analysis have also been used.

Case 55

A 19-year-old Nigerian student was seen in casualty complaining of breathlessness, aches and pains, and tiredness. A few days previously, she had a urinary tract infection for which she had been prescribed antibiotics. She told the casualty-officer that she had been diagnosed as a child at another hospital as having sickle-cell anaemia. She also said she had experienced a similar episode of breathlessness two years earlier after a termination of pregnancy. She was a non-smoker and apart from the antibiotics she was taking no other medication. On examination, she was clinically anaemic and breathless. Her blood pressure was 98/68 and her pulse was 96 beats/min. Emergency blood samples were taken and sent to the chemistry and haematology laboratories. The results of some of these tests are shown: haemoglobin 3.6 g/dl; white cells $17 \times 10^9/l$; platelets $190 \times 10^9/l$; reticulocytes were reported present. The chemistry results showed: sodium 136 mmol/l; potassium 5.2 mmol/l; urea 9.6 mmol/l; creatinine 0.13 mmol/l; bilirubin 88 μmol/l; alanine transaminase 46 U/l; alkaline phosphatase 223 U/l; lactate dehydrogenase 765 U/l.

Questions

1. What is the likely diagnosis?
2. What are the biochemical features of this disorder?
3. What are causes of an elevated plasma lactate dehydrogenase (LDH)?

Answers

1. This patient has a sickle-cell crisis. Broadly speaking, there are four main categories. This lady showed a haemolytic crisis with severe anaemia. Other manifestations include:

    (a) Vaso-occlusive crisis when blood hyperviscosity results in tissue hypoxia and infarction.
    (b) An aplastic or hypoplastic crisis due to bone marrow failure.
    (c) The sequestration syndrome which can lead to cardiovascular shock due to gross hepatic and splenic enlargement.

    Crises can be precipitated by many agents, including infection, hypoxia, operations and pregnancy.
2. As a result of poor tissue perfusion, there may be a metabolic acidosis with elevated plasma lactic acid. Impaired renal function can also result. Increased breakdown of erythrocytes causes an elevated plasma bilirubin concentration which is predominantly of the unconjugated form. There is increased urine urobilinogen and increased faecal stercobilinogen. The haemoglobin-binding protein, haptoglobin, is reduced in serum, due to the removal of the haptoglobin-haemoglobin complex by cells of the reticuloendothelial system.

Haemoglobin electrophoresis is used to show the structural haemoglobin variant. Sickling symptoms can occur in HbS homozygotes but also in some of the mixed haemoglobinopathies, such as SC, SD or sickle . cell-beta thalassaemia double heterozygote disease. Haemoglobin F can be elevated to between 5–15%.

Remember that patients with haemoglobin variants can show abnormal results for glycosylated haemoglobin determination which is used in the monitoring of glyaemic control in individuals with diabetes mellitus. As a result of chronic haemolytic anaemia, patients displaying sickle cell disease are more likely to have gall-stones.

3. The elevated plasma LDH in this patient is due to haemolysis and release of the enzyme from erythrocytes. Other haematological disorders can result in an elevation of plasma LDH such as the myeloproliferative diseases, leukaemias and pernicious anaemia. This enzyme exists as at least five different isoenzymes with different tissue specificities. Cardiac muscle shows predominantly the LD1 and LD2 isoenzymes and these increase in myocardial infarction. Skeletal muscle can show all the five isoenzymes and thus plasma levels of LDH can increase in various muscle disorders such as myositis. The LD5 isoenzyme is predominantly found in the liver and thus plasma elevations occur in a wide variety of hepatic disease. Many tumours also produce LDH, including lymphomas. Other conditions causing an elevated plasma LDH include hypothyroidism, pulmonary embolus or infarction, renal disease and acute pancreatitis.

Case 56

Tuesday was the day that the senior registrar in clinical biochemistry authorized the thyroid function results produced by the laboratory. Out of about 80 results, he pulled out three he wanted to make further enquiries about.

(1) The first result was that of an 80-year-old lady on the geriatric unit who was being investigated for carcinomatosis without a

known primary source. She was noticed to have been in atrial fibrillation and thyroid function tests had been sent to exclude hyperthyroidism. She was on medication, including analgesics and opiates. Her thyroid function test results were TSH 0.29 mU/l; fT3 4.3 pmol/l, and fT4 13.5 pmol/l.

(2) The second result was from a 49-year-old lady who complained of weakness and who had been seen in the medical out-patients' department. Her only medication was sleeping tablets. Thyroid function tests were ordered to exclude hypothyroidism. Her thyroid function tests showed TSH 7.5 mU/l and fT4 14.5 pmol/l.

(3) The third result was from a 32-year-old lady who attended the medical out-patients for treatment of her Hashimoto's hypothyroidism. She was on thyroxine treatment, at a dose of 150 μg day. She was taking no other medication apart from prothiaden for depressive symptoms. Her thyroid function tests showed TSH 10.4 mU/l and fT4 27.8 pmol/l.

Questions

1. In each case, give a possible explanation for the thyroid function results.

Answers

1. The first patient shows a low serum fT3 concentration, a normal fT4, and a TSH value within the reference range. These findings are consistent with a diagnosis of the sick euthyroid syndrome. Some patients, displaying illness that is not due to the thyroid gland itself, alter their peripheral conversion of thyroid hormones resulting in a low serum fT3. If measured, reverse T3 would be elevated in some cases. The normal TSH concentration implies that the patient is euthyroid. Sometimes, however, serum concentrations of TSH are also reduced. In severe non-thyroidal illness, fT4 serum concentrations may also be reduced. This is a prognostically bad finding and suggests a seriously ill patient.

   The explanation for these findings is poorly understood. In patients with non-thyroidal illness, it is recommended that thyroid function tests are repeated when the patient is better. In practice, this is sometimes not easy, but it is important as low thyroid hormones may mask thyroid disease. In an individual with a low TSH, one would need to exclude the rare T3 thyrotoxicosis, i.e an elevated serum fT3 with a suppressed TSH yet normal serum fT4 concentrations. Another source of diagnostic confusion occurs when fT4 and fT3 are both low due to non-thyroidal illness and the plasma TSH is low-normal. In this situation, the possibility of secondary hypothyroidism should be considered, i.e a pituitary or hypothalamic defect.

The second patient has an elevated serum TSH concentration but a low normal fT4 concentration. This would be in keeping with subclinical hypothyroidism, also known as compensated hypothyroidism. In these individuals, although there is a gradual deterioration in thyroid function, the thyroid gland is still able to release thyroid hormones in response to increasing pituitary stimulation via TSH. Sometimes these patients may show features of hypothyroidism. However, whether they should be treated with thyroxine is controversial. Nevertheless, they should be regularly reviewed, perhaps every few months, to establish whether their thyroid function tests have worsened. The serum TSH can become further elevated and the serum fT4 may decrease below the lower reference limit. Thus, overt hypothyroidism can occur, and annually a few percent of individuals show this trend, particularly if they have thyroid auto-antibodies.

At first sight, the thyroid results from the last patient may seem incongruous. Indeed, the doctor looking after this patient considered two possibilities, either a laboratory error or the very rare centrally mediated or secondary hyperthyroidism. This was based upon the logic that an elevated serum TSH was driving the thyroid gland to produce excess serum fT4. Similar results could also be a feature of tissue resistance to thyroid hormones. However, there is a much simpler and more likely explanation. The patient may have failed to take her thyroid replacement therapy except prior to her clinic appointment. This would result in a normal or high serum thyroxine concentration (hence an elevated fT4). However, the TSH would still be elevated because the pituitary gland has had insufficient time to respond to the short-lived thyroid hormone replacement. The patient eventually admitted that she had not regularly taken her thyroxine medication.

Case 57

A 45-year-old shopkeeper presented to the medical out-patients' department with swelling of his ankles. He had felt increasingly unwell over the past year and was experiencing tiredness and also nocturia. He was taking a calcium antagonist for hypertension, which had been commenced two years previously, and also warfarin, following admission to hospital with a left-leg deep vein thrombosis six months before his present appointment. He smoked 10 cigarettes per day and drank, on average five pints of lager per week. In his past medical history, he had undergone one operation five years previously for a perforated peptic ulcer and another 10 years previously for a ruptured appendix. He was married with two children who were both well and there was no evidence of any familial disorders.

On examination, his blood pressure was 164/94 and he had bilateral pitting oedema of his ankles and also sacral area. There was an early systolic murmur upon cardiovascular examination but he had no signs of cardiac failure. The rest of the examination was normal. In the clinic, a dipstick urine analysis showed the presence of protein, but no blood or glucose. Blood was taken for analysis and the following results were found: sodium 136 mmol/l; potassium 3.6 mmol/l; urea 17.4 mmol/l; creatinine 0.18 mmol/l; cholesterol 12.5 mmol/l; triglyceride 3.4 mmol/l; random venous plasma glucose 6.4 mmol/l; albumin 24 g/l; total protein 53 g/l.

Questions

1. What is the most likely diagnosis in this patient?
2. Suggest other biochemical tests which might have been performed in this patient.
3. Discuss the biochemical investigation of proteinuria.

Answers

1. This patient has a hyperlipidaemia, peripheral oedema, hypoalbuminaemia, hypoproteinaemia and proteinuria, which would suggest the nephrotic syndrome. Due to increased glomerular permeability, there is severe proteinuria. When the

loss of protein in the urine exceeds that being synthesized in the liver, then hypoproteinaemia results. The urine loss of protein is of the order of grams per day (often quoted as greater than 5g/24 hours), although it can be less than this.

As a consequence of the reduced osmotic colloidal pressure, fluid from the plasma enters the interstitial space. This can result in a reduced plasma volume with a subsequent increase in aldosterone secretion, leading in turn to a state of water and salt retention. Consequently, fluid accumulates in the interstitial space leading to oedema.

Also note that this patient has impaired renal function as evidenced by the moderately elevated plasma urea and creatinine. The recent past medical history of a thrombotic episode is also in keeping with the nephrotic syndrome, and is partly due to increased plasma fibrinogen. Similarly, there is increased hepatic synthesis of apolipoproteins resulting in hyperlipidaemia.

2. A timed urine collection, usually a 24-hour urine determination is clearly important in the diagnosing of the nephrotic syndrome. There are a number of causes of this syndrome, including glomerulonephritis, collagen vascular disease, diabetes mellitus, malignancies including multiple myeloma, infections, toxins and poisons. Serum C3 and C4 are useful determinants, and may be low in cases of immune-complex formation. Such complexes can damage the glomerular membrane. Streptococcal antibody studies may also be indicated. Another useful test is to study urine protein clearance ratios and to measure a selectivity index. The glomerular protein loss depends partly upon the size of pores within the glomerular membrane. By measuring the clearance of a large protein, such as IgG, and that of a small protein, such as albumin, and expressing this as a ratio, a selectivity index can be calculated. A low selectivity is seen in minimal change glomerulonephritis, whereas a high index suggests a non-selective protein loss.

3. When faced with a patient with proteinuria and having excluded a urinary tract infection, certain biochemical studies are indicated to explain its cause. Bence-Jones protein can be determined by urine protein electrophoresis with staining and immunofixation. This is seen in multiple myeloma and constitutes one of the overflow proteinurias, in which filtration of low-molecular-weight proteins through the glomerulus exceeds the normal reabsorption action of the renal tubules. Other

types of overflow proteinuria include myoglobinuria, haemoglobinuria, and lysozymuria.

The excretion of urinary albumin is useful in patients with diabetes mellitus. Here, low levels of albuminuria, so-called microalbuminuria, are predictive of nephropathy and also cardiovascular disease. Microalbuminuria is usually defined as an albumin excretion of between 30–300mg/24 hours on at least two or three occasions within a period of six months.

Remember that normal individuals lose less than 150 mg/day of protein in their urine. There is a condition called postural or orthostatic proteinuria in which there is increased proteinuria upon standing-up. However, normal proteinuria will be found in a sample taken just after a prolonged period of being supine.

In comparison to glomerular proteinuria, renal tubular proteinuria is also well described. This is due to a failure by the tubules to reabsorb protein. There is a tendency for increased excretion of low-molecular-weight proteins such as retinol-binding protein, $alpha_1$-microglobulin and $beta_2$-microglobulin, all of which can be measured in the urine. Urinary protein electrophoresis can also distinguish between tubular and glomerular proteinuria. Tubular proteinuria can be seen as part of the Fanconi syndrome, pyelonephritis, heavy metal poisoning, sarcoidosis and after ingestion of certain drugs, such as aminoglycosides (*Table 30*).

Table 30 Some causes of proteinuria

Reversible or benign forms	Due to fevers or exercise
	Postural
	Transient
Pregnancy	Functional
	Pathological, if severe
Urinary tract sources	Infections
	Tumours
Overflow types	Bence-Jones protein
Glomerular types	Nephrotic syndrome
	Glomerulonephritis
	Immune complex disease
	Diabetes mellitus
Tubular types	Fanconi's syndrome
	Renal tubular poisons

Case 58

A 41-year-old nurse was seen in the urology department because of a history of renal colic. A few months previously she had attended her general practitioner because of left-sided loin pain which had resolved after the administration of analgesics. On questioning, she admitted to recent abdominal 'cramps' and also constipation. She was a non-smoker and drank alcohol only rarely and she was not taking any medication. There was no notable family history. Examination showed a blood pressure of 138/88, no loin tenderness, and revealed no abnormalities. A plain abdominal X-ray showed a left-sided renal stone.

Blood was taken for biochemical analysis and the following results were obtained: sodium 140 mmol/l; potassium 4.1 mmol/l; bicarbonate 22 mmol/l; chloride 111 mmol/l; urea 8.7 mmol/l; creatinine 0.13 mmol/l; calcium 3.30 mmol/l; phosphate 0.55 mmol/l; magnesium 0.78 mmol/l; albumin 40 g/l; bilirubin 6 μmol/l; alkaline phosphatase 443 U/l; alanine transaminase 25 U/l; random venous plasma glucose 4.9 mmol/l. A 24-hour urine sample showed a calcium excretion of 9.4 mmol/l. In view of these results the urologist repeated the plasma calcium determination on an uncuffed venous sample. The result was 3.0 mmol/l, while a serum parathyroid hormone assay was 175 ng/l.

Questions

1. What is the most likely diagnosis?
2. What are the three main types of hyperparathyroidism?
3. What are other causes of urinary tract stones?

Answers

1. The most likely diagnosis is primary hyperparathyroidism. This patient shows a number of features of this condition. She describes symptoms of hypercalcaemia, such as constipation, abdominal pain and a urinary tract stone. She is also hyper-calciuric, with a urinary calcium excretion of greater than 8.8 mmol/l per 24 hours.

    The blood tests reveal an elevated serum parathyroid hormone (PTH) despite hypercalcaemia, which would normally be expected to suppress PTH levels. Note also the low plasma phosphate concentration sometimes seen in primary hyperparathyroidism, and also the mild hyperchloraemic acidosis, another described feature of the condition. This patient's renal function is also slightly impaired and she shows a high urinary calcium excretion. The other causes of hypercalcaemia are discussed elsewhere in this book (Case 12). Surgery was eventually decided upon as the best course of treatment, particularly in view of this lady's symptoms, renal stone, impaired renal function and the results of a bone scan.

Other useful investigations would include ultrasound studies of her neck to locate the abnormal parathyroid gland(s) and also a double thallium technetium isotope scan of the neck. Some centres use selective venous sampling and serum PTH assay to facilitate localization of parathyroid adenomas. It is also worth remembering the association with the multiple endocrine neoplasia (MEN) syndromes, which should be excluded.

2. Apart from primary hyperparathyroidism, there is the so-called secondary variety which has been defined as increased PTH production in response to a compensatory purpose. The compensatory stimulus is usually hypocalcaemia. Conditions associated with secondary hyperparathyroidism include chronic renal failure, malabsorption states resulting in vitamin D-deficiency, vitamin D-deficiency rickets, and pseudohypoparathyroidism. Sometimes, as a result of a long-term stimulus, the parathyroid gland(s) become autonomous resulting in an 'over'-secretion of PTH leading to a state of hypercalcaemia. This is called tertiary hyperparathyroidism.

3. There are many types of urinary calculi. The commonest type is the calcium oxalate stone, although calcium phosphate and calcium carbonate stones can also occur. The so-called triple stone is composed of magnesium-ammonium-phosphate and is associated with urinary tract infection. Other types of urinary tract stones include uric acid stones and those containing cystine, xanthine or fibrin. Uric acid stones and also the latter two are usually non-radio-opaque, unlike the other varieties.

There are many causes of renal stones. In about 25% of cases, the cause can be well defined and includes hypercalcaemia, hyperuricaemia, hyperoxaluria, infection by urea-splitting organisms, cystinuria, medullary sponge kidneys and distal tubule renal acidosis. Hyperoxaluria is worth further mention, as it can be a primary defect, either type 1 (glycolic aciduria) or type 2 (L-glyceric aciduria). It can also be the secondary variety, due to increased oxalate absorption from the gut as is seen in Crohn's disease, small bowel resection or malabsorption states. Other causes include a vitamin B_6 responsive form and diets rich in oxalate.

In many cases of urinary tract stones, there is not a well-defined cause, and the term idiopathic is used, even though hypercalciuria, hyperuricosuria or hyperoxaluria can sometimes be detected. In some cases, there may be low urinary concentrations of citrate, which is thought to inhibit stone formation. Idiopathic hypercalciuria still awaits an explanation, although in some cases there may be secondary hyperparathyroidism and increased intestinal absorption of calcium. More recent work has suggested the importance of reduced bone mineral content and high levels of monocyte interleukin-1 in this disorder.

In the investigation of urinary tract stones, urine (and if available stones) analysis for calcium, magnesium oxalate, cystine, phosphate and urate are useful. It is also useful to exclude a urinary tract infection, and to measure urine pH as uric acid and cystine tend to precipitate in low pH urine and calcium in alkaline urine.

Case 59

A 61-year-old retired estate agent was brought to casualty having collapsed at home one hour previously. His general practitioner made a diagnosis of myocardial infarction (MI) and had given him intramuscular diamorphine. He had previously suffered from angina for six years for which he had been taking isosorbide mononitrate and atenolol. Six months previously, he had a myocardial infarction but had recovered without any adverse effects. In casualty he complained of chest pain and shortness of breath. However, the ECG results were difficult to interpret, as they were not typical of a myocardial infarction, although there were ischaemic changes. Blood was taken soon after his arrival in casualty for biochemistry analysis and the following results were obtained: sodium 143 mmol/l; potassium 3.7 mmol/l; urea

5.7 mmol/l; creatinine 0.11 mmol/l; creatine kinase 233 U/l; aspartate transaminase 49 U/l; random venous plasma glucose 5.2 mmol/l.

Questions

1. Has the patient had a myocardial infarction?
2. What are the causes of an elevated serum creatine kinase apart from a myocardial infarction?
3. What other biochemical tests could be useful to confirm the diagnosis?

Answers

1. From the data presented here, one can not say categorically that the patient has had a myocardial infarction, although this is likely from the history. Creatine kinase (CK) is elevated, but in an acute myocardial infarction the plasma CK activity starts to rise usually within 3–6 hours, peaks at between 18–24 hours and returns to normal at about 72 hours. Creatine kinase activity usually increases by about 1000 U/l. The samples were taken at about one to two hours post-chest pain after the patient's collapse so it is possible that the blood sampling for CK activity was too early. The slight elevation of CK activity could be the result of skeletal muscle damage due to the patient's collapse and also the intramuscular injection of diamorphine. Blood sampling for CK activity should therefore be performed within the correct time-window from the suspected infarction or an alternative diagnostic test performed. Serial CK activity values compared against an action limit chart can help make the diagnosis of a myocardial infarction based upon a rate of change in plasma CK activity.
2. An elevated serum or plasma CK activity can be due to many factors. It is important to remember that there are three main isoenzymes: CK-MM is the predominantly skeletal muscle form and the main contributor to normal CK plasma levels; CK-BB is the brain isoenzyme; and CK-MB is the cardiac isoenzyme. Total CK activity can be increased in muscle damage, such as trauma, myositis, severe exercise, seizures, chronic renal failure and rhabdomyolysis. Both hypothermia and hyperthermia can similarly cause elevated levels, as can

alcoholism and hypothyroidism and hyperthyroidism. Certain tumours can produce creatine kinase and macro or complexed forms are present in some individuals, sometimes as the result of immunoglobulin-binding to the enzyme. Brain damage, whether due to trauma, cerebrovascular accident or tumours, can elevate total CK activity principally by elevating the CK-BB isoenzyme.

3. There is now increasing urgency to diagnose a myocardial infarction as early as possible because of the introduction of thrombolytic therapy. Ideally, this should be commenced as soon as possible after the event. This necessitates diagnostic tests which give both early and specific answers. The isoenzyme CK-MB is relatively cardiac-specific and peaks earlier than total CK activity at about 12 hours. Activity values of greater than .5% of the total CK activity are suggestive of a myocardial infarction, although very high values exceeding 25% may indicate the presence of a macro form.

Other tests that have been used with some success are determination of CK mass concentration (as opposed to CK activity) and also CK isoform determination. The rationale behind these tests is that they may offer greater specificity and/or sensitivity in making the diagnosis of a myocardial infarction. However, they still do not necessarily show early changes. Serum myoglobin (another muscle product) rises early after a myocardial infarction, sometimes within one hour after onset and in most cases by four hours, with a return to normal usually at about 36–48 hours. However, this test lacks specificity as elevation can occur in many forms of muscle damage.

At one time, before thrombolytic therapy added urgency, a myocardial infarction could be retrospectively diagnosed by taking serial blood samples and assaying not only for CK activity but also aspartate transaminase (AST) and lactate dehydrogenase (LDH). The former is not cardiac-specific, being also present in liver, kidney and erythrocytes, but after a myocardial infarction the AST activity peaks at between 24–36 hours and returns to normal at about 4 days.

Conversely, LDH activity peaks at between 12–24 hours after a myocardial infarction and returns to normal at about nine days, but this enzyme is present in many tissues including muscle, heart, kidney and erythrocytes. There are five isoenzymes of LDH; LDH1 and LDH2 are found in cardiac tissue and after a myocardial infarction LDH1 levels exceed that of LDH2. There has also been interest in the total CK:AST activity ratio which is said to be less than 10 in cases of myocardial damage.

All these tests have shortcomings regarding cardiac specificity and/or lack of early myocardial infarction diagnosis. Recent interest has centred upon serum troponin T determination. This supposedly cardiac-specific contractile protein starts to increase within a few hours of a myocardial infarction and stays elevated for several days.

Case 60

A 58-year-old factory worker was admitted under the care of the surgeons because of a recently diagnosed gastric carcinoma. He had initially presented to his general practitioner with weight loss and vomiting. A barium meal had suggested the presence of a gastric neoplasm. Unfortunately, on endoscopy the tumour was found to be ulcerated and partially obstructing the pylorus. However, an operation was considered possible as a palliative treatment to relieve the vomiting. On a recent ward-round, the hospital dietician had commented upon the patient's poor nutritional status. A routine pre-operation blood sample was sent to the chemistry department and the following results obtained: sodium 135 mmol/l; potassium 3.6 mmol/l; urea 4.6 mmol/l; creatinine 0.06 mmol/l; bilirubin 15 μmol/l; alkaline phosphatase 148 U/l; alanine transaminase 32 U/l; albumin 21 g/l; total protein 36 g/l. In view of these results, a 24-hour urinary protein collection was taken and showed a result of 246 mg/24 hour.

Questions

1. Give a possible explanation for the plasma albumin result.
2. What is the calculated plasma globulin concentration in this patient?
3. What further investigations could be performed to explain his plasma protein result?
4. This patient's plasma immunoglobulin concentrations were also shown to be low. Describe causes of hypogammaglobulinaemia in hospital patients.

Answers

1. A number of conditions are described in the literature as causes of hypoalbuminaemia (*Table 31*). Reduced synthesis of albumin can result from malabsorption states, malnutrition and poor protein intake, liver disease and some of the rare hereditary hypoalbuminaemic states, such as analbuminaemia. There can also be increased albumin catabolism, as is the case in hypercatabolic states including malignancy, severe trauma and hyperthyroidism. Another cause of a low plasma albumin is increased body loss, such as occurs in the nephrotic syndrome, from the gastrointestinal tract, exudates, burns and bleeding. Furthermore, there can be redistribution of albumin out of the plasma, as is observed in burns, sepsis and post-surgery. Haemodilution caused by inappropriate intravenous fluid replacement and also the physiological haemodilution of pregnancy can result in a low plasma albumin.

   This patient displays a number of possible causes of hypoalbuminaemia, including poor nutrition and malignancy. There is also a condition called protein-losing enteropathy. This can be associated with gastric carcinoma and can result in excess loss of protein from the gastrointestinal tract.

2. The calculated plasma globulin is equal to the total plasma protein concentration − plasma albumin concentration. In this patient, this comes to $36 - 21 = 15$ g/l.

Table 31 Some causes of hypoalbuminaemia

Albumin variants/abnormalities	Hypo- or analbuminaemia
Protein loss	Protein-losing enteropathy
	Nephrotic syndrome
	Exudates and transudates including burns, bleeding,
Reduced synthesis	Malnutrition
	Hepatic disease
	Malabsorption
Increased albumin catabolism	Trauma
	Sepsis
	Carcinoma
	Surgery
	Hyperthyroidism
Redistribution of albumin	Haemodilution
	Burns
	Pregnancy

3. A diagnosis of protein-losing enteropathy can be made by radiolabelling studies, using for example labelled albumin which can be given by intravenous injection. A four-day stool collection is then made and greater than 2% loss in the stool is suggestive of protein-losing enteropathy. A less invasive technique is to measure faecal alpha$_1$-antitrypsin which is elevated in protein losing enteropathy. In low protein states, the nephrotic syndrome should be excluded by a urinary protein determination (which is only slightly elevated in this patient). It is also useful to quantitate plasma immunoglobulins to see if a secondary hypogammaglobulinaemia is present. This patient was eventually shown to have a protein-losing enteropathy.

4. Hypogammaglobulinaemia can be primary or secondary. Primary conditions can show selective immunoglobulin deficiency, such as the isolated IgA deficiency which occurs in 1 in 500 members of the population. Other disorders can involve all classes of immunoglobulin, such as is seen in severe combined immune deficiency (SCID) or X-linked agammaglobulinaemia (Bruton's syndrome). There are also rare forms of immunodeficiency associated with ataxia telangiectasia or thrombocytopenia.

The secondary causes of hypogammaglobulinaemia include those conditions resulting in excessive protein loss, e.g. nephrotic syndrome or protein-losing enteropathy. Other causes include bone marrow disorders and myotonic dystrophy. It is said that IgG is predominantly lowered in these diseases. Conversely, severe infections, uraemia and lymphomas produce a secondary immunodeficiency affecting mainly IgM.

Index

Made in the USA
Monee, IL
07 July 2026

56552254R00095